Lose It!

Lose It!

THE PERSONALIZED
WEIGHT LOSS REVOLUTION

Charles Teague and Anahad O'Connor

RODALE

© 2010 by FitNow, Inc.

Rodale books may be purchased for business or promotional use or for special sales. For information, please write to: Special Markets Department, Rodale Inc., 733 Third Avenue, New York, NY 10017.

Printed in the United States of America
Rodale Inc. makes every effort to use acid-free ⊗, recycled paper ♻.

Book design by Christina Gaugler

Illustrations courtesy of Lose It!
Photographs by Thomas MacDonald/Rodale Images

Library of Congress Cataloging-in-Publication Data

Teague, Charles.
    Lose it! : the personalized weight loss revolution / Charles Teague and Anahad O'Connor.
        p.   cm.
    Includes bibliographical references and index.
    ISBN 978–1–60529–094–2 pbk.
    1. Weight loss.   2. iPhone (Smartphone)   I. O'Connor, Anahad.   II. Title.
RM222.2.T43   2010
613.2'5—dc22   2010041063

Distributed to the trade by Macmillan
2   4   6   8   10   9   7   5   3   1   paperback

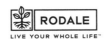

We inspire and enable people to improve their lives and the world around them.
www.rodalebooks.com

To everyone who is out there Losing It!

CONTENTS

FOREWORD BY GRETCHEN RUBIN,

author of *The Happiness Project*

A few years ago, I decided to embark on a "happiness project." I spent a year test-driving the wisdom of the ages, current scientific studies, and lessons from popular culture to see what worked. If I did all the things I'd always intended to do and followed the advice I'd heard over the years, could I actually become happier? I didn't make a dramatic upheaval to my daily routine—just little changes, here and there. When the year was over, I was surprised by how easily I'd changed my life without changing my life. I really did manage to make myself happier.

I organized my happiness project around resolutions—everything from "Quit nagging" to "Make my bed" to "Sing in the morning" to "Keep a one-sentence journal" to "Imitate a spiritual master."

My happiness project convinced me that resolutions—kept faithfully—can make a huge difference in contributing to happiness. If you want to make a positive change in your life, a very effective strategy is to figure out what resolutions to make and how to keep them. Keeping the actual resolution will boost happiness, of course, but even apart from that, the sense of growth, of having made a vow to yourself and stuck to it, the sense of self-mastery . . . all these things are enormously satisfying.

The challenge is that, no surprise, it's fun and easy to make a resolution, but it's very challenging to keep a resolution. Something like 44 percent of Americans enthusiastically make their New Year's resolutions—I know I always do—but many of us make and break the same resolution year after year; in fact, about 80 percent of resolution makers abandon their resolutions by mid-February.

Year after year, one of the most popular resolutions (along with other perennials like "quit smoking" and "spend less") is the resolution to lose weight. Alas, about two-third of dieters gain back the weight they've lost within the year.

These facts are pretty discouraging. Does that mean it's pointless to make resolutions? I don't think so. You can't succeed unless you try.

But if you really want change, you have to think about it, plan it, probe it, keep yourself accountable, and have a plan—just reflexively saying "This year I'm really going to eat healthy" won't make it happen.

Having tried and failed to uphold many resolutions myself, I'm fascinated by the question of what allows people to keep resolutions. Why does one person decide to drop 20 pounds and manages to do so without much fuss, while another person battles those same 20 pounds for decades? Why does one couch potato suddenly decide to start going to the gym and then works out regularly for years, while another couch potato just can't get off the couch?

One key to sticking to a resolution, it turns out, is to hold yourself accountable. The constant review of your resolutions, and the knowledge that you are being held accountable to them, makes a huge difference. So how do you hold yourself accountable? Here are some useful strategies:

1. **Frame your resolution in concrete actions.** If you resolve to "Eat more healthfully" or "Lose weight," it's hard to hold yourself accountable. It's easier to be answerable for a specific action, like "Eat five servings of

vegetables and fruit every day" or "Bring my own lunch to work four days a week."

2. Be accurate. When you're trying to do something like lose weight, it's important to know how much, and how many calories, you're eating. Studies show that people tend to underestimate dramatically both the portion size and calorie content of their food, but to change what you're eating, you have to know what you're eating.

3. Keep a chart. Having made a resolution, you have to check yourself in some way. Keeping a written record is an excellent way to keep yourself honest and mindful; a chart acts as a reminder that allows you to keep your resolution active in your mind and to mark your progress. Also, seeing what you've achieved in the past is a powerful source of motivation for the future. Give yourself those gold stars!

4. Join with other people. Even more useful than keeping a chart is knowing that real, live people are cheering you on—and holding you accountable. Also, research shows that we enjoy activities more when we do them with other people.

5. Commit to an action. Studies show that taking an action, like signing a pledge or registering for a program, will help you hold yourself accountable for your resolutions. People who are trying to make life changes such as losing weight are more likely to succeed when they tell others what they're doing.

Lose It! is an excellent tool that makes it quick and convenient to combine all these strategies.

With Lose It! you can easily track the food you eat and the calories you consume every day—no more airy guesses. "Well, nuts are healthy, so it's probably okay to eat as many as I want." "Gosh, I haven't eaten much today, I don't think, so I deserve a brownie. Maybe two brownies. Okay, three." "I pick up dinner at my favorite fast-food place a few times a week, and that's probably . . . what? About 400 calories a shot?" Lose It! reminds you what you've eaten and tells you the consequences, so you can make choices that support your resolutions.

Making better choices adds up over the long haul. We often overestimate what we can get done in a short amount of time—"I'm going to lose 8 pounds in 2 weeks!"—and underestimate what we can get done over a long period, by making small changes—"I'm going to lose 30 pounds this year."

By keeping you accurate and accountable, Lose It! makes it easier to stick to your diet—or even better—eventually to give up food monitoring all together. We all want to reach a point where we eat healthfully, automatically, every day, without being "on a diet."

Mindfulness is one of the keys to happiness, which is unfortunate for me because I'm not a very mindful person. But the Lose It! program can help anyone develop mindfulness while eating because it prompts us to pause, to think, and to appreciate our food.

Founding Father Benjamin Franklin is a patron saint for people trying to keep a resolution. During his life, in addition to signing the Declaration of Independence, investigating electricity, inventing bifocals, founding one of the first volunteer firefighting departments, and acting as ambassador to France, Franklin kept a chart of the thirteen qualities he wanted to cultivate. Once a day, he'd score himself on whether he'd observed such virtues as "temperance," "silence," "industry," and "frugality." Of this chart, he observed, "though I never arrived at the perfection I had been so ambitious of obtaining, but fell far short of it, yet as I was, by the endeavor, a better and a happier man than I otherwise should have been had I not attempted it."

While no book or mobile application can ensure that we'll stick to our resolutions perfectly, they can help us to do better. And by doing better every day, we can work our way to healthier and happier lives.

INTRODUCTION

You're holding this book in your hands because you want to lose weight, so let's get right to it.

Short of surgical intervention, there's no way you will ever strip away fat without abiding by one immutable law of nature that's as true today as it was 1,000 years ago: You have to burn more calories than you eat. At the end of the day, there's not a diet on Earth that can help you lose weight unless you obey this fundamental truth.

So why waste your time with trendy foods and crash diet plans that promise quick results—that vanish just as quickly—when you can lose weight on your own terms? With *Lose It!*, you create a strategy that's tailored to *your* lifestyle and includes the foods *you* want to eat.

All you need to get started is a little information: the number of calories that you burn in a day. Your calorie needs are as unique to you as your DNA, and your plan for losing weight should be, too. Once you have this all-important number, you will know exactly how much food you can eat while achieving your dream of a new, sleeker you.

Of course, therein lies the problem. Most Americans have no idea how many calories they're consuming, and they *certainly* don't know how many calories they burn in a day—and the cost of ignoring this crucial information is nothing short of staggering. According to health authorities, average adult men and women burn an estimated 1,800 to 2,200 calories a day. And yet studies show that Americans have a per capita consumption of 3,790 calories a day. That's enough extra calories to gain more than 10 pounds every month! The list of health problems that often accompany all those extra pounds is also sobering: heart disease, hypertension, stroke, type 2 diabetes, back pain, and more.

By now you're probably wondering, *How many extra calories am I taking in?*

Before you venture a guess, keep in mind that a nationwide study conducted in 2010 found that 63 percent of Americans have no idea what that number is, and most of us grossly underestimate our calorie intake.

That's where this book comes in.

In November of 2008, Lose It! was launched as a free mobile application that offered users the ability to track the calories they eat as well as the calories they burn in *real time,* allowing them to see exactly how food and exercise impact their weight. It distilled weight loss down to its very essence—calories in versus calories out—but unlike other weight-loss plans, it allowed users to create their own personalized strategies for success. With Lose It!, users could eat what they wanted and could access their calorie budget and food and exercise logs at the touch of a button.

Since its debut, more than 6 million people have downloaded the app (it's one of the most popular free downloads in the App Store), and tens of thousands of people follow Lose It! via social media. Through the simple quest to make losing weight as easy as possible, a revolution began.

The ecstatic reviews and success stories on iTunes, the testimonials on loseit.com, and the comments on the Lose It! Facebook and Twitter pages all testify to the fact that this program not only works, but it also makes the daunting task of losing weight feel manageable, and even enjoyable.

This book, in addition to offering the very latest information on the science of weight loss, incorporates data collected from millions of users of the Lose It! app, as well as the very best tips and strategies provided by those who've lost weight successfully—whether they lost 10 pounds or more than 100 pounds. In the following pages, you'll find everything that you need to know to be in control—once and for all—of your weight. There are no hard-and-fast rules. With *Lose It!,* you get the tools you need to create a plan that works for you and you only. As any of the millions of people who have already lost weight with the app will tell you, *Lose It!* puts control over food and exercise squarely in your hands. You make the rules, and you're responsible (and accountable) for the results.

So how do you create your own weight-loss plan?

Using your height, weight, age, and a few other pieces of personal data, you'll determine how many calories you burn in an average day. Once you've decided how much weight you want to lose and how quickly you want to drop it, you'll calculate a daily calorie budget that will get you to your goal weight within your desired time frame.

Though you don't need to use the free mobile app or log onto the Lose It! Web site to benefit from this book, tracking your calories, exercise, and progress digitally in conjunction with reading this guide will allow you to check your budget at any second of the day so you always know exactly how you're doing. And many of the graphs and charts available online can help you uncover the behavior patterns and habits that are affecting your progress.

Whether you're standing in line at Quiznos and deciding between the Baja Chicken sub and the Honey Bacon Club or wondering if you have room in your daily calorie budget for a McDonald's Extra Value Meal, all you need to do is pull out your phone or mobile device to look up the calorie count and see how much you've already consumed for the day. There's no need to agonize over food decisions because there's no mystery about what you're eating.

What if you're getting close to your calorie limit for the day but you're still hungry? Maybe you have only 200 calories left and you're craving a particularly satisfying 300-calorie meal. The solution is simple: Add more calories to your budget. Spend 30 minutes walking around your neighborhood or engaged in any other activity that burns 100 calories—you'll find many more options in this book. Suddenly, you have 100 additional calories to spend on whatever you choose. Finding the motivation to break a sweat is a lot easier when you know those negative calories are giving you some much-needed room to eat the foods you love.

The more you learn to think about food and exercise as energy—calories consumed and calories burned—the more you will begin to instinctively think about food from an economic standpoint. As you track your meals and accumulate a log of your own personal data, you'll quickly realize which foods give you the most bang for your calorie buck and which splurges just aren't worth it. Before you know it, making smarter choices becomes a habit, and your body and your health will reflect the results of those decisions.

Think about it: How much easier will your life be when you eliminate the guesswork surrounding food? You'll always know what's on your plate, and nothing beats the satisfaction of knowing you ate foods you enjoyed and *still* lost weight.

The Lose It! philosophy is based on five crucial pillars.

1. **Embrace mindful empowerment.** Just say no to extreme diets! Take control of your body and the foods you put in it. Empower yourself

with the knowledge of your unique calorie needs and the facts that will help you to make smarter choices at every meal.

2. **Track your calories.** All you have to do is track one single variable: calories. There are no points or complicated algorithms to follow. Just keep track of what you eat and be diligent about it. (Snacks count!) Even if you think you know how many calories you need every day and the number of calories in the foods you've been eating, you're likely to be shocked when you see your daily tally.

3. **Track your habits.** As you log your foods over time, you'll begin to spot behavior patterns and habits—good and bad—that you can modify to help you meet your weight-loss goals. As you learn from your behavior, you can personalize your experience and make the changes that work for you.

4. **Track your exercise as negative calories.** Use exercise as a way of staying within the parameters of your calorie budget for the day, no matter what you eat. Overindulge by 100 calories? Then spend 10 more minutes jogging on the treadmill. You'll also learn how to burn more calories in less time to get the most benefit out of your gym sessions and discover the simple, everyday activities you can do to torch extra calories. (Here's a hint: Spend less time sitting!)

5. **Benefit from peer support.** You can lose it alone, but losing it with friends will boost your odds of success. Peer support motivates and inspires you, keeps you accountable, and provides insight from those who have been there, done that. The Lose It! app brings social support into the 21st century, with instantaneous interaction at your fingertips, either through the app or online. Need some help refraining from a 3 a.m. ice cream binge? Go online and find a friend who will talk you out

of it. Worried you might go overbudget one too many days in a row? Share access to your budget with a sibling or your spouse: If he or she sees that you're slipping, you'll get a swift reminder that helps you get right back on track.

(((())))

If you're tired of being unhappy with your weight but you're equally tired of following someone else's rules for how to shed pounds, you've finally found the key to your success. This book will give you the tools to create a sustainable, realistic weight-loss plan that works for you now and will continue to work for years to come. Unlike other diets, this is a plan that won't abandon you when you hit your goal weight. Lose It! will help you maintain your weight loss and stay healthy *for life*.

The time to Lose It! is now, and everything you need is right in your hands.

Chapter One

Mindful Empowerment

Calories Unmasked

For many years, we've been taught that in order to lose weight we have to learn to live without the foods we love. To get lean, you have to be extreme . . . right?

Wrong. Scientific research consistently shows that this approach doesn't work—and your epic battle with the bathroom scale proves it. Dieting is a zero-sum game. You can lose weight fast by cutting out certain foods and learning to live with cravings, but more than one-third of people on typical diets regain all of the weight they lose within a year. Long-term studies of Americans who've dropped 30 or more pounds and have kept it off for a minimum of 1 year—and in some cases, decades—offer proof that drastic change is not the answer. The people who are able to lose weight and maintain their weight loss successfully aren't following 30-day diet plans or subscribing to meal delivery services. They don't eliminate carbs or fat, and they *certainly* don't skip meals.

They all follow a strategy that worked long before the Era of the Diet, and one that will work long after the last fad diet is gone.

They reduce calories and they exercise.

If this bit of information doesn't come as a surprise to you, then here's something that might: You can do it, too. Lose It! will help you reach your health and fitness goals, and if you ask any one of the millions of people who've already benefited from this revolutionary weight-loss tool, they'll attest to the fact that you don't have to suffer for your success. If nothing gives you more satisfaction than a pillow-soft loaf of bread fresh from the oven (like quite a few Lose It! users), then don't give up your beloved carbs! If a hot dog with the works is your ultimate weakness, no one's going to stop you from indulging.

There are millions of reasons why Lose It! will work for you—about 6 million, in fact. That's because more than 6 million people have used the program since its inception. Each one has been able to create a *personalized* plan, tailored to his or her unique schedule, lifestyle, dietary needs, and food preferences. Lose It! simply empowers them with knowledge—the knowledge of how many calories they should be eating and how many calories they really are eating. This knowledge gives them (and you) the power to make small changes that add up to major losses.

The best possible weight-loss plan, after all, is the one that you design yourself. Just ask Brian Newby of Florida, who cycled on and off of the Atkins Diet for years, struggling to stay on the plan because he simply couldn't say no to bread. (For Brian, an Alabama native, a meal isn't a meal if it doesn't come with biscuits.) Then Brian discovered Lose It! After a year of following the program dutifully, he's lost more than 100 pounds—and he didn't have to give up the carbs he loves. Another Lose It! pro, Blaine Smelscer of Texas, shrunk himself from 280 pounds down to 180—without giving up the hot dogs, burgers, and chicken fingers that form the foundation of his diet. He simply learned how to adjust his portion sizes and choose burgers, dogs, and chicken with fewer calories.

With Lose It!, you can forget about following someone else's idea of what you should and shouldn't eat and simply learn to love food again. One of the first things you'll discover is how to calculate a calorie budget that reflects your specific needs. When you stay within its limits, you're in the Green Zone. But when you eat more calories than you've budgeted for a day, you will enter the Red Zone—dangerous territory. It's similar to your financial budget. When you see how much you're spending on your choices (some of them regrettable), you'll learn to plan ahead and spend wisely. The end result? You'll spend on the things you really want—and stay in the green.

"I'm teaching myself to eat better," said Sabrina Euton, who lives in Georgia and has lost more than 40 pounds since January of 2010. "I know it's called Lose It!, but for me it's a tool that I use to teach myself to treat my body better. I can't tell you the last time I ate fast food. I used to pick up food on the way home from work all the time. Now I buy food and portion it into individual servings so I'm able to come home, pull out one container, and heat it up. I'm still eating things I want to eat. I'm just scheduling and preparing them ahead of time. My husband and I don't have that last-minute, 'What are we going to have for dinner?' fight anymore. Our local pizza shop was always the winner of that fight. They knew us by our first names."

THINK ECONOMICALLY, NOT JUDGMENTALLY

From now on, what you choose to eat is between you and your taste buds. A study by Tufts University scientists, published in the *Journal of the American Medical Association,* showed that people who followed weight-loss plans that they didn't perceive as being too restrictive lost more weight and lowered their risk of developing cardiovascular diseases more than those who felt deprived. Simply put, the freedom to eat the foods you like can mean the difference between keeping the pounds off for good and finding yourself shopping for the next size up in a few short months.

When you consider that 70 percent of Americans surveyed in a 2010 study said that they were concerned about their weight, and nearly 80 percent said that they wanted to either lose or maintain their weight, the nationwide need for a little food freedom becomes more than clear.

But here's the scary part: Most Americans have *no* idea how many calories they're consuming and where those calories are going! The same 2010 study—carried out by the International Food Information Council Foundation—found that only 12 percent of Americans could correctly estimate the number of calories they should be consuming in a day based on their age, weight, height, and activity level. And nearly half of all Americans have no idea how many calories they burn in a day.

It's not that they aren't trying to eat less and burn more. A majority of Americans say that to lose the weight, they're changing the amount of food they eat and the amount of time they spend being active. But making those changes without any knowledge of the amount of calories you need and the amount of calories you're burning daily is like driving across the country without a map. There's a chance you'll reach your destination, but there's also a chance you'll take a wrong turn and end up in Seattle when you were shooting for San Diego.

The premise of the plan is simple: The more you know about the number of calories you need to burn to reach your target weight and the number of calories that are in the foods you like to eat, the smarter the choices you make will be. To lose weight without depriving yourself, you need to know precisely how many calories you can afford to spend. When you ignore this basic information, the calories add up faster than you can say, "spare tire."

You wouldn't walk into Saks Fifth Avenue and buy a coat off the rack without peeking at the price tag, would you? And you certainly wouldn't take that coat to the register without having a rough idea of what's in your bank account. Yet most Americans go on a caloric spending spree every time they open up their fridge or walk into a sandwich shop.

ANOTHER ONE BITES THE DUST

Even if you think you're pretty careful about what you eat, there's a good chance you're consuming more calories than you realize. A 2006 study by scientists at Cornell University and published in the *Annals of Internal Medicine* found that the more food you have on your plate, the more likely you are to underestimate the number of calories it contains (in some cases, by as much as 40 percent!). Tack onto that all of the little snacks and bites you sneak between meals each day, and it's no wonder the weight won't take a hike.

Yup, that's right. Those little bites add up, and they affect us all—the parents who finish their kids' mac 'n' cheese and uneaten chicken nuggets, the stealthy snacker who sneaks a spoonful of ice cream every night before bed, the sampler who always grabs those bite-size bits of free muffins at the local coffee shop, and even the human garbage disposal who makes a habit of putting away those last bites of hamburger or cheese lasagna that his friends have left stranded on their plates.

Plate Cleaning, Parenting Pounds, Sneaky Snacks, and Small Bites—They All Add Up!

If You Ate	That Equals	How Often	That Adds Up To	Total Weight Gain
2 chicken nuggets from your kid's plate	84 calories	5 days a week	420 calories	0.5 pound a month, or 6 pounds a year
1 bite of mac 'n' cheese from your kid's plate	30 calories	5 days a week	150 calories	0.2 pound a month, or 2.4 pounds a year
1 spoonful of Häagen-Dazs Chocolate Chocolate Chip ice cream just before bed	75 calories	6 nights a week	450 calories	About 0.5 pound a month, or about 6 pounds a year
1 free muffin sample on a toothpick at your coffee shop	About 41 calories	3 days a week	123 calories	About 0.1 pound a month, or 1.7 pounds a year
The last 2 bites of your buddy's cheese lasagna	About 139 calories	Twice a week	278 calories	About 0.3 pound a month, or 3.6 pounds a year
10 Goldfish crackers from your kid's lunch bag	30 calories	4 times a week	120 calories	More than 0.1 pound a month, or 1.6 pounds a year
A handful of french fries from a friend's plate	53 calories	Twice a week	424 calories	0.5 pound a month, or 5.8 pounds a year
A bag of Nacho Cheese Doritos from the vending machine	250 calories	Twice a week	500 calories	More than 0.5 pound a month, or 7 pounds a year
That last bite of your kid's peanut butter and jelly sandwich	51 calories	Twice a week	102 calories	More than 0.1 pound a month, or 1.4 pounds a year

You're about to learn how easy it is to track all of those calories you've been eating and forgetting about the second they hit your gullet. As millions of successful Lose It! users have discovered, the more you know about your individual choices and preferences—past, present, and future—the better equipped you'll be to judge when you can get away with a must-have splurge and when you're better off going with an alternative that tastes good but won't break the bank (the calorie bank, that is). And sometimes you may even choose to skip the splurge altogether to ensure that you stay securely in the Green Zone.

21ST-CENTURY CALORIE COUNTING

At this point you're probably wondering, What's with all the the fuss over calories? Isn't it a chore? Do I have to lug around a pencil and notebook everywhere I go? Wasn't calorie counting a thing of the '80s?

Yeah, and so were cassette tapes. Thirty years ago we counted calories using pen and paper, just like we listened to mix tapes on a Walkman. It's not that we don't listen to music anymore, we just have a new and more efficient way of doing it: We go online and download songs onto a portable device we can fit into our pockets. Counting calories with Lose It! works similarly; think of it as iTunes for weight loss. Ask any member of the Lose It! community—it's *that* revolutionary.

We're living in the 21st century. Technology has made almost every aspect of our lives easier, from communication to cooking. So why not use your smart phone, Blackberry, or iPod to help you lose weight?

Modern technology has given us tools that make losing weight less of a struggle, but the Lose It! app is based on time-honored, scientifically proven methods that have been around for decades. And you know what? Keeping track of your foods with a pen and paper is just as effective today as it was 20 years ago. If that's your preference, you can still benefit from this book. It's all about creating a strategy that works for you— whether you keep a paper journal or use a more modern device, any method you use to track your calories will help you reach your goal. The important thing isn't how you track, it's that you track diligently—every bite, every day.

As a nation, we need calorie counting now more than ever. We've all been consuming foods that are enormously energy-dense but not particularly filling or healthy. As the Centers for Disease Control and Prevention (CDC) reported a few years ago, the percentages of carbs and fat in the national diet are constantly rising and falling, shifted by the ever-changing winds of the diet industry. First the "fat is evil" trend caused people everywhere to abandon even the healthiest fats and encouraged them to eat more carbohydrates; then the nationwide anticarb frenzy changed all that. But the one common denominator that's been tied most directly to our country's outward expansion has nothing to do with fat or carbs. We weigh more because we're eating more.

There's no doubt that nutrients play a significant role in the calorie game. Studies show that fiber keeps us full and protein triggers the release of hormones that curb hunger, while diets high in simple carbs spawn the hunger-inducing insulin spikes that propel us toward the kitchen. But at the end of the day, what pushes the needle on the scale in the wrong direction is eating too many calories (of any kind), and what matters most is not the breakdown of nutrients in the nationwide caloric pie, but the fact that the pie itself keeps getting bigger and bigger and bigger.

The tagline of the last couple of decades may as well have been: "It's the calories, stupid," because it's been calories all along. From 1971 to

2000, calorie intake increased in direct proportion to our ballooning waistlines. Calorie consumption grew nearly 10 percent for men and roughly 20 percent for women. Is it any coincidence that the national obesity rate has *doubled* since the 1970s? Today, more than two-thirds of Americans are overweight. Clearly it's time for a calorie-counting comeback.

Each of us is responsible for the choices we make every day, but there's plenty of blame to go around. It's clear, for instance, that the hand that feeds us has become increasingly generous. Over the past 30 years, restaurant portion sizes have grown so large that we've lost all track of what a normal, healthy portion should look like. We've also fallen hook, line, and sinker for clever marketing tactics. Many "healthy-sounding" restaurant dishes are actually calorie catastrophes. Order a Carolina Chicken Salad at Ruby Tuesday and you'll be eating the caloric equivalent of two Big Macs— a calamitous 1,157 calories. Go with the Grilled Chicken Salad (547 calories) or the Turkey Burger (699 calories) and you're *still* getting more calories than a Big Mac. Even some of the "Fit & Trim" options, like the Herb Crusted Tilapia, which comes with broccoli, mashed potatoes, and 662 calories, blow a Big Mac out of the water. Amazingly, you're better off skipping these seemingly sensible choices altogether and just going with Mickey D's classic old-school double burger.

Concerned about the epidemic of weight-related diseases like type 2 diabetes and the millions of dollars in health care that will be needed to treat overweight Americans, our government has finally taken action to protect us from marketing gimmicks and help us make better food choices. Now more than 200,000 fast-food and other chain restaurants—specifically, restaurants with 20 or more locations—are required to post calorie counts on menus, menu boards, and drive-throughs. The law applies to vending machines, as well, and restaurants and vendors can face criminal penalties if they don't comply. How's *that* for calorie control?

At the same time that restaurants are being held accountable, the FDA is taking on food manufacturers by tackling the widespread problem of deceptive labeling and calorie counts on food packages. The agency announced in early 2010 that it wanted food manufacturers to make two crucial changes: Move calorie counts from the back of food packages to the front (where they're far more visible) and stop putting impossibly small serving sizes on the labels (so people aren't duped into consuming more calories than they realize). The food labels on this and the opposite page offer three examples of these ridiculously small serving sizes. One bottle of Vitaminwater, according to the label, has 2.5 servings. Have you ever bought a bottle of Vitaminwater, drunk less than half of it, and then finished off the rest over two other occasions? When was the last time anyone ate two Fig Newtons or exactly 15 chips?

If you're worried that these changes mean Big Brother is telling you what to eat, think again. Just like Lose It!, these regulations are actually designed to give the power back to you, allowing you to make food choices that are right for your waistline—not the food industry's bottom line. In

Vitaminwater

Nutrition Facts	
Serving Size 8 fl oz (240 mL)	
Servings Per Container 2.5	

Amount Per Serving	
Calories 50	

	% Daily Value*
Total Fat 0g	0%
Sodium 0mg	0%
Potassium	†
Total Carbohydrate 13g	4%
Sugars 13g	
Protein 0g	

Vitamin C 120%	•	Vitamin B_3 40%	
Vitamin B_6 40%	•	Vitamin B_{12} 40%	
Vitamin B_5	•	Magnesium †	
Zinc 10%	•	Chromium 10%	

†Not a significant source of calories from fat, saturated fat, trans fat, cholesterol, dietary fiber, vitamin A, calcium and iron

* Percent Daily Values are based on a 2,000 calorie diet

Fig Newtons

Nutrition Facts

Serving Size 2 cookies (31g)
Servings Per Container About 13

Amount Per Serving

Calories 110	Calories from Fat 20

% Daily Value*

Total Fat 2g	3%
Saturated Fat 0g	0%
Trans Fat 0g	
Polyunsaturated Fat 1g	
Monosaturated Fat 0g	
Cholesterol 0mg	0%
Sodium 130mg	5%
Potassium 75mg	2%
Total Carbohydrate 22g	7%
Dietary Fiber 1g	4%
Sugars 12g	
Protein 1g	

Vitamin A 0%	•	Vitamin C 0%
Calcium 2%	•	Iron 4%
Phosphorus 0%	•	Magnesium 0%

* Percent Daily Values are based on a 2,000 calorie diet. Your daily values may be higher or lower depending on your calorie needs:

	Calories:	2,000	2,500
Total Fat	Less than	65g	80g
Sat Fat	Less than	20g	25g
Cholesterol	Less than	300mg	300mg
Sodium	Less than	2,400mg	2,400mg
Potassium		3,500mg	3,500mg
Total Carbohydrate		300g	375g
Dietary Fiber		25g	30g

Lay's Potato Chips

Nutrition Facts

Serving Size 1 oz. (28g/About 15 chips)
Servings Per Container 11

Amount Per Serving

Calories 150	Calories from Fat 90

% Daily Value*

Total Fat 10g	16%
Saturated Fat 1g	6%
Polyunsaturated Fat 4.5g	
Monosaturated Fat 4.5g	
Trans Fat 0g	
Cholesterol 0mg	0%
Sodium 180mg	7%
Potassium 330mg	9%
Total Carbohydrate 15g	5%
Dietary Fiber 1g	4%
Sugars 0g	
Protein 2g	

Vitamin A 0%	•	Vitamin C 10%
Calcium 0%	•	Iron 2%
Vitamin E 6%	•	Thiamin 2%
Niacin 6%	•	Vitamin B_6 4%
Phosphorus 4%	•	Magnesium 4%

* Percent Daily Values are based on a 2,000 calorie diet. Your daily values may be higher or lower depending on your calorie needs:

	Calories:	2,000	2,500
Total Fat	Less than	65g	80g
Sat Fat	Less than	20g	25g
Cholesterol	Less than	300mg	300mg
Sodium	Less than	2,400mg	2,400mg
Potassium		3,500mg	3,500mg
Total Carbohydrate		300g	375g
Dietary Fiber		25g	30g

fact, recent studies have found that these calorie postings don't cause people to turn around and walk away from the fast-food counter. In essence, we can still have our burgers and eat them, too. But we can also save a few hundred calories in the process.

New York City has required chain restaurants to post calorie counts since April of 2008. In 2010, researchers at Stanford University published a study analyzing more than 100 million Starbucks transactions that occurred between January of 2008 and February of 2009. This allowed them to see precisely how the new postings affected people's purchasing patterns. As control groups, they used Starbucks locations in Boston and Philadelphia, where there were no calorie postings.

The study found that at the Starbucks locations in New York City, the average calories per transaction dropped by a relatively modest 6 percent, but that people who habitually bought high-calorie foods changed their habits far more than the average customer. These folks (and you know who you are, pastry lovers) lowered their calories per transaction by an average of 26 percent. Perhaps most interesting is that it wasn't beverage transactions that were affected—most people still ordered their usual lattes and macchiatos. Much of the reduction in calories came instead from changes in food purchases.

So what gives?

Most of us go to Starbucks primarily for a caffeine hit, but once we're at the counter and we see those beautiful pastries in the gleaming glass case, it's easy to fall for a muffin. Or a brownie. Or a scone. How bad could one scone be, right? Turns out a single blueberry scone will cost you 460 calories and a seemingly healthier choice, the zucchini walnut muffin, will cost you even more: 490 calories and nearly half a day's worth of fat (44 percent, based on 2,000 calories a day).

In other words, the Stanford scientists say, while we're unlikely to change our order for the 370-calorie Mocha Frappuccino we came in for—a decadent snack in its own right—we *are* likely to sacrifice that blueberry scone we just noticed in the pastry case—a calorie-laden afterthought.

That's not depriving yourself. That's just being smart.

IT'S NOT AN EMPTY CALORIE IF IT FILLS YOUR ENERGY GAP

So what happens if you buy the scone anyway?

How will your body treat that delicious dose of 460 calories? Well, it depends. A calorie is simply a unit of energy, and your body needs calories for fuel, both for exercise and to maintain basic bodily functions such as respiration, digestion, and circulation.

Most people don't realize it, but your body burns a tremendous amount of energy while at rest. It's sort of like looking down at New York City from the window of an airplane thousands of feet in the air: From a distance, everything appears calm and orderly, but on the ground, there's a whirlwind of frenetic activity. When you're lying on the couch with a remote in your hand, your body burns a surprising amount of energy just to keep your lungs going, your brain functioning, and your blood and heart pumping. You're even burning calories by reading this book.

Your weight remains stable as long as the number of calories you consume doesn't exceed the number of calories your body burns. As the balance shifts in one direction or the other, it creates an energy gap—a change in your body's energy balance point—causing you to either lose or gain weight. This gap can be a surplus or a deficit. For instance, if you've had nothing to eat all day, then you'll have an energy deficit, and a bite of that scone—which is mostly carbs, fat, and sugar—will be put to good use. Of course, an apple or a nutritious sandwich would be a better choice, but strictly speaking, those seemingly "empty" calories will be metabolized and used to fill your energy gap.

So while eating a scone isn't the issue, per se, the problem is that most of us don't eat a scone to fill an energy gap. We buy it because it's

SURPRISING WAYS YOU BURN CALORIES DOING THE MOST MUNDANE ACTIVITIES

(30 minutes of each, unless noted otherwise)

Activity	125-pound person	155-pound person	185-pound person
Sleeping	19 calories	23 calories	28 calories
Watching TV	23 calories	28 calories	33 calories
Reading this book, seated	34 calories	42 calories	50 calories
Brushing your teeth (5 minutes)	12 calories	15 calories	18 calories
Playing with your kids (moderate effort)	120 calories	149 calories	178 calories
Food shopping, pushing a cart	105 calories	130 calories	155 calories
Standing in line	38 calories	47 calories	56 calories
Cooking	75 calories	93 calories	111 calories
Having sex	120 calories	148 calories	194 calories
Taking a stroll (without the dog or children)	86 calories	107 calories	128 calories

Source: The Harvard Heart Letter, July 2004

right in front of us and it tastes good. Far too often that scone becomes a means of excess calories that go beyond what our bodies require. It takes 3,500 calories to make 1 pound of body fat. Even if you typically burn everything you consume (through mundane activities), you only need to eat one blueberry scone every day for roughly a week to move

HOW MANY SCONES A WEEK WILL ADD A POUND A MONTH?

One blueberry scone is 460 calories.	A pound of fat is 3,500 calories, so roughly 8 scones will pack on a pound. (3,500 ÷ 460 = 7.6)	One month is about 30 days, or 4 weeks.	Thus, all it takes is two scones a week to pack on 1 pound a month. (8 scones ÷ 4 weeks = 2)

the needle on your scale one unit to the right—that is, to gain a pound (see the chart above to crunch the numbers).

But let's say that you're one of those people who sees calorie counts posted next to each tempting item and decides not only to avoid the scone, but also to order your Frappuccino without the 2 tablespoons of whipped cream (100 calories) that you'd normally have. Then, over the course of 35 days, you'll become 1 pound lighter. Make five small changes like this, and *you'll lose 5 pounds in the next month!*

WHAT'S THE BIG DEAL OVER 50 CALORIES?

When you consider the scope of the obesity crisis in America, it's easy to blame some of our most outrageous eating habits for our extra pounds. We are, after all, a nation that buys pizza by the foot at Little Caesars and the Double Down (a bunless sandwich made from two slabs of fried chicken with bacon and cheese layered in the middle) at KFC. But surprisingly, when scientists looked closely at our eating habits, they found that the average American—the key word here being "average"—consumes about 50 more calories a day than he or she expends.

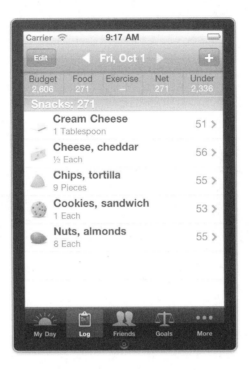

The average American consumes about 50 more calories a day than he or she expends—a seemingly trivial amount but more than enough to pack on the pounds.

That certainly doesn't sound like much. But over time, those routine calorie surpluses add up. This is why long-term studies show that the average adult in the United States gains between 1 and 2 pounds every year. Before you shrug off 2 annual pounds or even a single pound, consider that over a decade that will result in a gain of 10 to 20 pounds—literally the weight of a Bridgestone spare tire.

Of course, this is just an average weight gain. Many of us go far beyond an excess of 50 calories. No surprise, then, that according to the CDC nearly 33 percent of Americans are overweight and another 34 percent are

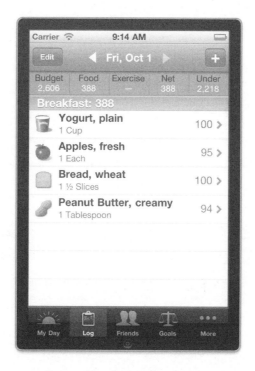

**Cut out just 100 calories a day,
and in one month you'll lose almost a pound.**

so overweight that they're classified as "obese." On top of that, another 6 percent are classified as "extremely obese."

So altogether, about three out of four adults are taking in too many calories. In some cases, the excess is slight; in others, it's excessive. But we can take solace in the fact that we're not alone. Slow and steady energy gaps are being documented in every corner of the globe. In Scotland, a recent decade-long study found that only 20 percent of the adult population remained at a stable weight during the 10-year period, while nearly half of the population gained more than 10 pounds and 18 percent gained more than 20. A pound-a-year increase has been documented in Australian women, and a 1.5-pound-a-year jump has been recorded in Chilean women. And yet another study, this time in health-conscious Sweden, revealed a 7.3-pound increase for women and an 11-pound increase for men during a 17-year period.

Scientists say these international trends in weight gain are due to minute energy gaps, on the order of 30 to 100 calories—meaning the average person is taking in 30 to 100 more calories a day than he or she is burning.

In a report published in 2009, a joint task force of health experts and obesity scientists declared these small energy gaps a major problem, saying: "The available data suggest that many populations are gradually gaining weight, which is being fueled by a relatively small difference between energy intake and energy expenditure. Put simply, on average, most people are consuming only slightly more calories than they are expending and, consequently, are gradually gaining weight at an average of 1.1 to 2.2 pounds per year."

But the flip side of this slow and steady weight gain is that it can be easily reversed. If instead of eating an extra 50 calories a day you *cut* 50 calories a day, you would gradually lose weight. These small and entirely manageable and nonrestrictive changes are responsible for the amazing results of Lose It! community members. And what's even more impressive (and so simple) is that if you were to cut 500 calories out of your day, every day, you could lose an entire pound each week—without making dramatic changes. All you have to do is learn about your eating patterns and assess what you can change. There may be one obvious source of a few hundred calories that you could eliminate, whether it's a blueberry scone, the bread that comes with your soup, or the cookie (or two) you have after lunch.

The Usual Suspects: 500 Calories You Can Easily Eliminate Every Day

Blueberry Muffin from Dunkin' Donuts	510 calories
Meat Lover's Pan Pizza from Pizza Hut (1 slice)	480 calories
Cinnamon Chip Scone from Panera Bread	530 calories
Vanilla Triple Thick Shake from McDonald's (16 ounces)	550 calories
Grande Peppermint White Chocolate Mocha Espresso from Starbucks (made with whole milk)	500 calories

This is entirely doable. In fact, according to the joint report, 90 percent of weight gain in the United States could be stopped simply by cutting out just 100 calories a day. That's a couple slices of Kraft American cheese. You can eliminate that many calories a day by skipping a bag of Lay's potato chips, using fat-free milk instead of cream in your coffee, ordering your burger without the cheese and mayo, or walking instead of taking the bus.

We've all been inundated with the idea that weight loss can be achieved rapidly by making drastic changes. But successful, sustainable weight loss—the kind that lasts a lifetime—is all about altering your habits. And this is why millions of people in the Lose It! community have been able to shed so many pounds. As we'll discuss in the chapters that follow, Lose It! gives you the most effective and innovative tools available to get to the bottom of your own eating habits. Only when you know yourself—and your personal pitfalls, preferences, and routines—can you truly get on track with a weight-loss solution that will help you succeed. (And it will not be the same solution for that guy on the treadmill beside you or the woman sitting next to you on the bus.)

So, are you ready to join the personalized weight-loss revolution that's changing the way America sheds pounds? The first step is to get to the bottom of how many calories you're eating every single day and then compare that with how many you should be consuming.

CALCULATING YOUR DAILY BUDGET

The first thing you'll need to do is calculate your own personal daily calorie budget. So how do you figure it out?

Well, if you've already downloaded Lose It! for your phone—free of charge, of course—then we'll do it for you. All you have to do is enter a few stats: your height, weight, gender, and age. If you already have the app, you can skip to page 22.

LET THE WEIGHT LOSS BEGIN

Getting started with Lose It! is simple and free. Just go online and visit loseit.com and follow the instructions to set up your *free* account. You can also find the free Lose It! app in the iTunes App Store; just search for "Lose It!"

If you've never used the app or the Web site, here are a few simple steps that will let you figure out your calorie budget on your own. Fair warning: This will involve a little bit of math. But don't worry—you don't need an advanced degree in calculus to figure it out. Just find a calculator and let's get started.

To begin, you'll use a simple equation that was developed by nutrition scientists. It's called the Mifflin Equation, and it measures your resting metabolic rate, or RMR. This is a measurement of the energy your body requires at rest—literally the energy you would burn if you were sprawled on the couch with a remote control in your hand.

The Mifflin Equation requires your weight in kilograms (which you can calculate by dividing your weight in pounds by 2.2) and your height in centimeters (which you can calculate by multiplying your height in inches by 2.54).

For men, the equation is as follows:

$$5 + 10(weight) + 6.25(height)—5(age) = RMR$$

For women, it's only slightly different:

$$10(weight) + 6.25(height)—5(age)—161 = RMR$$

So for a 30-year-old man who stands 5 foot 8 (172.7 centimeters) and weighs 180 pounds (81.8 kilograms), it would look like this:

$$5 + 10(81.8) + 6.25(172.7)—5(30) = 1,752\ RMR$$

In the second step of the calculation, you multiply that RMR value by your Physical Activity Level, or PAL, which is the amount of activity you get in a normal day, excluding exercise. Your personal activity level refers to all those mundane activities that burn calories but don't include *actual* exercise. (We exclude exercise here because that's something that you add in later.)

The average person—say, a typical office worker—has a PAL value of about 1.45, which corresponds to a fairly light level of activity. (This is the value you're assigned when you use the app.) You can use this value, if you like. But if you have a far more physically demanding job—such as working in a daycare center where you chase around after kids all day, or have to do any kind of physical labor that requires strength and stamina—then you should select a higher PAL because you burn more calories in an average day than someone who sits at a desk and stares at a computer screen. Below are the PAL values. Choose the one that best reflects your lifestyle most days of the week.

<1.40 = Very inactive (someone who is very immobile)

1.40–1.69 = Sedentary (typical office worker with infrequent exercise)

1.70–1.99 = Moderately active (construction worker or office worker who exercises 5 days a week)

2.00–2.40 = Extremely active (person who exercises 2 hours daily)

Once you've chosen a PAL value, multiply that number by your RMR to get your daily calorie needs. For example, let's say that the 30-year-old male mentioned above who had an RMR of 1,752 has a PAL of 1.7.

1,752 x 1.7 = 2,978 calories

His daily calorie needs are roughly 2,978 calories.

REMEMBER: SLOW AND STEADY WINS THE RACE

Now that you've determined your calorie needs, you can set a budget to help you achieve your desired weight.

Let's say that you discovered that you burn about 2,500 calories in a typical day (without exercise). Your goal, just for the sake of simplicity, is to lose a very conservative 10 pounds in 10 weeks. Remember: 1 pound is about 3,500 calories; 3,500 × 10 = 35,000. So in order to reach your goal, you'll need to accumulate an energy (calorie) deficit of 35,000 calories over the next 10 weeks. Now let's break that down into more attainable values: That's 3,500 calories a week, or roughly 500 calories a day.

In other words, since you typically burn 2,500 calories a day, you'd have to stay 500 calories *below* that number each day to lose 10 pounds in 10 weeks. So you'd want to set a budget that keeps you at or below 2,000 calories a day, which would mean you'd be consuming 500 *fewer* calories a day than you're burning. Over the course of 10 weeks, that budget of 2,000 calories—if you stuck to it—would get you to your target weight (70 days × 500 calories = 35,000 calories, or 10 pounds). You could achieve this either by cutting back on calories alone or by cutting back some calories and adding exercise to your daily activities. Either way, you'll be increasing your negative calorie balance.

For health reasons, Lose It! recommends that you lose no more than 2 pounds a week. If you're using the app, it's automatically set at this limit. It's a vastly different approach from all of those diet plans that promise you'll lose 5, 10, or even 15 pounds in the first week. Remember, the average person gains about 2 pounds in an entire year and up to 20 pounds in a decade. Trying to lose a decade's worth of weight in 1 week just isn't realistic. Sure, you can do it, but it requires drastic measures that aren't sustainable over the long haul. (It's also not much fun to eat salads for every meal.) As a study published in the *New England Journal of Medicine* in 2006 pointed out, most people who start a diet take about 1 year to regain one-third of the weight they lost, and most of them are right back where they started in 3 to 5 years.

Drastic measures are exactly why most diets fail. Remember, slow and steady wins the race. Take it from Donneen Kelley Parrott, a Lose It! user who has lost more than 40 pounds since September of 2009 and has *kept it off* with little effort. Donneen, who's 40 years old and lives in Oklahoma, has struggled with her weight her entire life and tried "everything under the sun," from the Atkins Diet to Slim-Fast.

"Mostly my problem was a lack of motivation," she admits. "Diets just aren't realistic; I was always hungry. When you force yourself to drink [meal replacement] shakes three or four times a day or eat something that you don't really want, then once you hit your goal you're just going to return to what you were eating before and gain the weight back."

With Lose It!, Donneen didn't drink every meal or force herself to eat foods she didn't like. And she wasn't convinced this new strategy was going to work.

"I was skeptical when I first used Lose It!," she admits. "I wasn't sure that I could eat this many calories and still lose 2 pounds a week."

But it worked. And it wasn't difficult. One of the easy changes she made was swapping her meals at McDonald's with meals from Subway.

"A Happy Meal from McDonald's is almost 500 calories by itself. You can easily consume 2,000 calories at a fast-food restaurant without even thinking. I used to eat the value meals, but those are almost 1,000 calories. I don't go to McDonald's anymore. There are only two fast-food restaurants I eat at now: Subway and KFC. I can still go to McDonald's, if I want to, but I know that I can get twice as much food from Subway for the same number of calories."

For Donneen and so many others in the Lose It! community, it's the small changes that matter most. Weight loss is about taking incremental steps in the right direction and realizing that each of those steps—like eating a 6-inch Meatball Marinara sandwich at Subway for lunch instead of heading to McDonald's for a Quarter Pounder—gets you closer to your goal.

SETTING YOUR BUDGET WHILE MAKING ROOM FOR DATE NIGHT

Once you've determined how much weight you want to lose and how many calories you need to slash from your day to get there, you can start to make those small but important changes. Again, let's use the metaphor of your calorie budget as your financial budget. When you're budgeting your hard-earned dollars, the first things you need to make sure you have covered are the essentials: mortgage payment or rent, food, water, and electricity. Then you have your discretionary purchases, like movie tickets, dinners out, new clothes, and the occasional vacation. With a calorie budget, you should also plan for (and spend on) the essentials. Ideally, breakfast, lunch, and dinner should consume 70 to 80 percent of your calorie budget. Discretionary calorie purchases—snacks, sodas, and desserts—should account for no more than 20 to 30 percent of your budget.

This allocation of calories works for most people and is likely to keep you feeling satisfied all day long—even if you break down your three big meals into several smaller meals. For example, Lose It! user Jennifer Mueller Krause of Washington, who's lost more than 40 pounds since 2009, says she's a "grazer." She prefers to eat a snack or small meal every couple of hours to give herself the energy she needs to keep up with her young daughter. She eats energy-boosting snacks throughout the day: a hard-boiled egg with a side of steel-cut oats; a tortilla stuffed with Canadian bacon; a small sandwich made with whole wheat bread, Laughing Cow cheese, and a little meat; a handful of apple slices and grapes; or a bowl of Greek yogurt topped with agave nectar and sliced strawberries and bananas.

They may be "snacks," but they account for about 75 percent of her daily calories—her "meal" calories. The rest of her calories are spent on splurges like an Iced Caffè Mocha with whipped cream at Starbucks. So while Jennifer doesn't stick to a traditional meal structure, she *does* stick to her daily calorie budget and has been able to lose weight successfully by creating an individualized plan that works for her lifestyle.

Cara Griffin of California, who has lost more than 100 pounds using Lose It!, also makes her own rules. She doesn't think about the percentage or breakdown of snacks in her budget—she simply eats dessert when she's in the mood for it and can spare the calories. If she's spent all of her calories on meals, then she doesn't eat snacks or desserts. But if she has a few hundred calories to spare, she knows she can treat herself to the things she wants. It's a vastly different approach from the diets she's tried in the past.

"For me, Lose It! is more realistic than diets. If I want some candy or cookies, I still eat them, I just work them into my calorie budget. I can still eat the foods that I want, just in moderation."

There's no one "right" way to spend your calories; the important thing is to create a structure that works for you. The goal is to lose weight without depriving yourself, and no one knows what strategy works best for you better than you do. Millions of people have started right where you are today, and with the help of Lose It!, they've made lasting, meaningful weight loss a reality.

HOW SMALL CHANGES CAN HELP YOU LOSE 100 POUNDS

Not long ago, Blaine Smelscer found himself staring down at the scale in his doctor's office, frightened by the number he saw.

Like many Americans who struggle with their weight, the self-employed father of two had spent years shuffling from one diet to another. Blaine would lose 10, 20, maybe even 30 pounds at a time, but eventually all of the weight he'd lost would come back—and then some. Blaine, who lives in Texas, comes from a super-size family that takes pride in their super-size appetites.

"We love food," he says. "Fried food, greasy food, hamburgers, pizza, fried chicken . . . anything like that."

But growing up on comfort food had some uncomfortable consequences. At his high school graduation in 1994, Blaine carried over 200 pounds on his 5-foot-10 frame. And as he got older, he only got bigger.

Finally, while standing on the scale in his doctor's office, he saw a number that shocked him: 280 pounds. His blood pressure was dangerously high and his blood sugar and cholesterol levels were also soaring. A devoted family man with a loving wife and two small children, Blaine knew he needed to take better care of himself. His doctor sat him down and offered some advice that would change his life.

"He said, 'There's a good application on the iPhone that can help you lose weight, and it's pretty simple. It's called Lose It!,'" recalls Blaine.

So Blaine pulled out his phone and downloaded Lose It! right there in the office. He started tracking his foods over the next several days and learned how many calories he'd been taking in. Like a lot of guys, he'd assumed his caloric intake—even with his love of hot dogs and burgers—was about average.

He could not have been more wrong.

As it turned out, Blaine was easily consuming between 3,000 and 5,000 calories a day. He was stunned, but there was no denying the numbers. Lose It! brought him face-to-face with his habit of overeating—on some days by an inch, and on others by a mile.

"I started learning about serving sizes, and that's when I realized how much I overate. Once I learned that, I started fixing meals with fewer servings that still fill up my plate."

Blaine was ready to take another shot at weight loss. But this time, he wasn't going to deprive himself of the foods he loved or expect rapid results. He wasn't going to abolish carbs or swap steaks for salads. With the help of Lose It!, he was simply going to train himself to eat good food in healthy quantities.

He set a goal of losing 50 pounds. Using Lose It!, he created a budget of 2,200 calories a day—less than he was used to, but still plenty of room to eat comfortably. And Blaine could easily keep track of his daily progress and his distance from the Red Zone. He was literally able to see, morsel by morsel, that he was in control of his own weight loss.

"I love hot dogs," he says, "especially Oscar Mayer beef franks. But I started eating Oscar Mayer 98 percent fat-free turkey hot dogs instead, so I went from 130 calories a serving down to 40. Fast-food hamburgers would be 200-plus calories for a Quarter Pounder, whereas you can get extra-lean hamburger at the grocery store for 130 calories a serving, so that cuts it almost in half.

"I also switched to extra-lean turkey, which has only 120 calories in 4 ounces. Skinless chicken breasts or skinless chicken tenderloins are only like 100 calories for 4 ounces, too. And you can find fat-free Ruffles potato chips that have half the calories of the regular ones—80 calories instead of 160."

In addition to shopping smarter and cooking more often, Blaine also made lower-calorie choices when he went out for a meal, and he learned to pace himself when he ate.

"When I do go out, I've learned what I can eat that will fill me up but cost me fewer calories. And I take my time now and eat slowly. I used to eat just to get stuffed, and then when it was mealtime again, I'd eat even if I were still full. Now I know I'm supposed to eat just until I start to feel full, not to stuff myself. When I feel satisfied, I stop eating. Later on in the day, I'll wait until I'm hungry to eat again."

Blaine didn't realize it at the time, but he was adopting a habit that has long been a custom in Okinawa, an island off the coast of Japan. This island is home to one of the healthiest populations on Earth—a group of people who also enjoy the greatest longevity of any population in the world. Okinawans practice a form of appetite and calorie control called "Hara hachi bu," which means that you eat until you are 80 percent full; then you stop. When you pace yourself, you allow your stomach enough time to tell your brain that it's reaching its limit. Ultimately you walk away from the table having ingested fewer calories.

Pacing himself helped Blaine consume smaller meals. He also redistributed how he spent his calories throughout the day so that he always felt full, instead of bingeing, letting his hunger build to the point where he was ravenous, and then bingeing again.

When Blaine reached his weight-loss goal of 50 pounds, he went back to his doctor for a checkup, and he was given a clean bill of health. His blood sugar and cholesterol levels were in the normal range, and he no longer needed blood pressure medication. Today, Blaine has lost more than 100 pounds and has no intention of regaining the weight.

"This is a lifestyle change that I've made, and I have no reason to go back to the old way," he says proudly.

Chapter Two

The Power of Paying Attention

Tracking Calories and Losing Weight, One Meal at a Time

Here's a simple question: How many times a day do you think about food?

Take a moment to really consider your answer. It's not something most people usually stop to think about.

Like many people, you probably eat at least a few solid meals a day, so that's three food decisions right there. Throw in some snacks, then toss in a few cups of coffee, soft drinks or other drinks, and for good measure add a few more meals to account for weekend splurges, and we're easily talking about at least a dozen food-related decisions every day.

Does that sound about right to you?

Actually, it's far from it.

According to scientists at Cornell University, the average person makes more than 220 food-related decisions *every single day*.

No, that's not a typo. In an average day, you make hundreds of food decisions, many of them small ones that take only seconds. Do I grab a handful of M&M'S as I walk by my colleague's candy bowl? Do I get that blueberry scone with my coffee at Starbucks? Do I help myself to a bagel from the spread in the conference room or a piece of coffee cake at the PTA meeting?

Every one of those decisions, as inconsequential as it may seem, is far more important than you realize. Each and every one of them is a chance to do something that could either benefit you in your efforts to trim pounds from your stomach or push you closer and closer toward a lifetime of sucking in your gut every time you zip up your jeans.

The Lose It! weight-loss revolution takes place one meal at a time. Just imagine if you took only a fraction of all the food decisions you make in a single day and made a conscious effort to turn them into smarter choices. You could save yourself hundreds if not thousands of calories a day and ultimately say "so long" to those stubborn pounds that won't seem to budge.

Ask any longtime Lose It! user and they'll tell you that they lost the weight—and have kept it off—because Lose It! arms them with the knowledge to make informed decisions when it comes to these 200-plus daily choices.

Let's go back to our Starbucks dilemma from Chapter 1, since it's one many of us often face. To scone or not to scone? What if you said, "No, I don't need the 460-calorie scone, but I *will* get a Marshmallow Dream Bar that's *less than half* the calories so I don't feel deprived and overeat something else when I get home"?

If you made that decision 5 days a week when you walked into Starbucks for your afternoon pick-me-up, you could easily dodge some unwanted pounds.

If you swapped a Marshmallow Dream Bar (210 calories) for a Blue-berry Scone (460 calories) every weekday you went to Starbucks, you'd save . . .

   After 1 week: 1,250 calories, or about 0.4 pounds

   After 1 month: 5,000 calories, or about 1.4 pounds

   After 1 year: 60,000 calories, or about 17 pounds

   After 2 years: 120,000 calories, or about 34.3 pounds

   After 5 years: 300,000 calories, or about 85 pounds

THERE ARE NO TRICKS HERE

The Starbucks scone example is powerful proof that small changes can add up to big weight loss. Saying "no" to a scone could keep you from gaining 17 pounds over the course of a year. (That's assuming you're not giving in to other high-calorie food decisions, of course.)

But let's say you don't go to Starbucks and you don't eat scones. The same principle still applies: There are plenty of times each day that you're presented with an opportunity to make a smarter food decision that won't undermine your efforts to lose weight. Lose It! empowers you to think economically—not emotionally—about food, which allows you to comparison shop for your calories. In the same way that you might have an emotional attachment to a Ferrari ("This car will make me happy!"), a look at your budget and some comparison shopping would help you real-ize that you could make yourself just as happy with a more economical choice. When you're faced with a food decision—whether at Starbucks, in the supermarket, or while standing in front of your refrigerator—Lose It! will help you override your instinctive, short-term emotional thinking ("This food will make me happy!") with practical knowledge.

Think about it: If we all devoted this much consideration to our more than 200 food choices every day, then our nation as a whole probably wouldn't be in the midst of a growing obesity crisis. (Remember, scientists have found that 90 percent of all weight gain could be stopped if we all cut our daily calorie intake by only 100 calories.) In this chapter, you're going to learn how to become a more mindful eater—you'll become someone who knows how to save calories at every meal by making choices that support your long-term goals, rather than giving in to emotional impulses.

The sooner you figure out where you've been wasting calories— that is, the places where you could easily make smarter choices and lower-calorie substitutions—the sooner you can start to lose weight. And there's only one way to know how much you've been consuming and how you can start making smarter choices, and that's by tracking your calories. There are no ifs, ands, or buts here: Tracking and logging your foods is at the very core of the Lose It! philosophy, a tried-and-true strategy that will help you master the calorie game. So let's get started.

TRACKING YOURSELF RIGHT INTO WEIGHT LOSS

As mentioned in Chapter 1, you can keep track of the foods you eat each day using pen and paper, or to keep track electronically, download Lose It! to your mobile device or log onto loseit.com.

Now, you may be thinking, "I don't see how writing everything down— or tracking it electronically—can make that much of a difference." Well, consider this: In 2008, a study in the *American Journal of Preventive Medicine* found that the simple act of keeping a food diary can *double* your weight loss. The study, which was carried out at several clinical research centers around the country over a period of more than 2 years, tracked nearly 1,700 overweight or obese adults, all of whom were encouraged to cut back on calories and exercise moderately. At the end of the study, they had all benefited from these strategies; however those who kept a food journal 6 or 7 days a week lost an average of 18 pounds in the first 6 months, compared with 9 pounds in the group that didn't track their foods.

"The more food records people kept, the more weight they lost," said Jack Hollis, the lead author of the study and a researcher at Kaiser Permanente's Center for Health Research in Oregon. "It seems that the simple act of writing down what you eat encourages people to consume fewer calories."

Of course, it's not just the act of keeping a log that helps you lose weight—it's what that log reveals that really makes a difference. There is something truly stunning about seeing in black and white just how many calories you've consumed over the course of a single week, or even over the course of a single day, and where, in particular, those calories have come from. Most of us have only a rough idea of how many calories we consume, and we all tend to have a selective memory, especially when it comes to the foods that we'd like to forget: the spoonfuls of Oreo topping added to your frozen yogurt, the extra dollop of sour cream piled on a burrito, the three bites of mac 'n' cheese you cleaned off your kid's plate. As soon as they're down the hatch, it's as if they never crossed your lips. Keeping a food log allows you to identify patterns and see cold, clear calorie counts that will motivate you to make easy changes that might not otherwise occur to you.

That's exactly what happened for Nicole Comer Jones, a 26-year-old mother of two in Alabama. Nicole found herself weighing more than 200 pounds after having her second child. She considered herself a health-conscious eater, and yet, at 5 foot 4 and 208 pounds, she was

(continued on page 38)

KEEPING A FOOD DIARY

Downloading Lose It! is the quickest and simplest way to keep track of your foods, but if you prefer pen and paper, here are a few tips to get you started.

1. In the front of a pocket-size journal or notepad, draw a chart with the foods you eat most frequently. Use the rest of the notebook as your food journal, and refer to the chart when you log the calories of the foods you eat most often.

2. Use a separate page for each day, and divide the page into four vertical columns—breakfast, lunch, dinner, and snacks—to make a simple chart. At the top of each vertical column, note the meal or time of day you ate; in each of the boxes underneath the columns, note the food consumed and the number of calories it contained. (See pages 36 to 37 for an example.)

3. Make sure you keep track of everything, even small snacks and bites throughout the day, so you know exactly where your calories are coming from. Keep track of portion size, too.

4. At the end of the day, add up all the calories you've consumed. If you're over your limit, look for places where you're taking in unnecessary calories—and most important, be honest with yourself. It's the only way you'll be able to eliminate the sources of extra weight.

Sample Log
Date: Thursday

Breakfast 8:30 am	Calories	Snack 11:00 am	Calories	Lunch 1:00 pm	Calories	
Scrambled Eggs (2 whole eggs)	200	Nature Valley Oats 'n Honey granola bar	95	Oven-roasted Boar's Head turkey (2 slices)	60	
Oscar Mayer Real Slices Bacon (3 slices)	210	Dannon Light & Fit Nonfat Yogurt (Strawberry)	80	Kraft American Singles (1 slice)	60	
Wonder Bread (white, 2 slices)	190			Hellmann's mayonnaise (1 Tbsp)	100	
Tropicana orange juice (8 fl oz)	110			French's Yellow Mustard (1 tsp)	0	
Maxwell House Original Blend coffee (10 fl oz)	2			Lettuce, generic (1 large leaf)	0	
				Tomato, raw (2 slices)	21	
				Lay's Sour Cream & Onion chips (17 chips)	160	
				Coca-Cola (12 fl oz)	140	
	712		175		541	

Snack 4:00 pm	Calories	Dinner 7:00 pm	Calories	Total
Rold Gold Classic Style Tiny Twists (17 pretzels)	110	McDonald's Premium Southwest Salad with Crispy Chicken	430	
Red Delicious apple (1 apple)	80	Coca-Cola, medium (21 fl oz)	210	
		McDonald's Hot Caramel Sundae	340	
	190		980	2,598

overweight. After downloading Lose It!, she was floored to discover that she was eating close to 3,000 calories a day.

"It blew my mind," she says. "I started logging my food and was shocked to see how much I really was eating. I thought I was doing pretty good. But when I looked at my numbers, I was amazed. Most people don't realize what they put in their mouths every day."

By logging her foods, Nicole was able to spot some patterns that were causing her to pack on the pounds. One of the most surprising calorie traps she discovered was something she never would have suspected: skim milk. Nicole was adding it to everything, from cereal to protein shakes, causing her to drink about a gallon of skim milk on most days.

"Because it's skim milk, you think it's harmless," Nicole says, "But actually it has a lot of calories and a lot of carbs and sugar."

Nicole immediately made some changes. In addition to cutting down on her overall milk consumption, she also switched from skim milk to a lower-calorie option that she loves: almond milk.

"It tastes very good, and it has more protein and fewer calories," she says.

Once she saw the impact of this one change, she was motivated to uncover more calorie traps and make similar adjustments to her diet. Within months, she'd lost 40 pounds.

The chart on the opposite page shows you some simple ways you can cut calories every day without missing out on any of the foods you love. Keep in mind that if you made just half the changes listed in this chart (without altering any other parts of your life), you'd lose more than 10 pounds in a year!

Hold the Mayo!

Try these small changes that offer big results.

If You Like Using This	Then Switch to Using This	And You'll End Up Saving	Do It 5 Times a Week and You'll Save	After 1 Year That's
Fat-free milk, 86 calories per cup	Almond Breeze Original, 60 calories per cup	26 calories per cup	130 calories	6,760 calories, or about 2 pounds
Mayonnaise, 103 calories per 2 Tbsp	Nonfat mayo, 11 calories per 2 Tbsp	92 calories per 2 Tbsp	460 calories	23,920 calories, or 6.8 pounds
Table sugar, 15 calories per packet	Truvia (sweetener), 0 calories	15 calories per packet	75 calories	3,900 calories, or 1.1 pounds
Grey Poupon Savory Honey Mustard, 20 calories per 2 tsp	French's Classic Yellow Mustard, 6 calories per 2 tsp	14 calories per 2 tsp	70 calories	3,640 calories, or about 1 pound
McDonald's Creamy Ranch Sauce, 170 calories per serving	McDonald's Tangy Honey Mustard Sauce, 60 calories per serving	110 calories per serving	550 calories	28,600 calories, or 8.2 pounds
McDonald's Southwestern Chipotle Barbeque Sauce, 60 calories per serving	McDonald's regular Barbeque Sauce, 50 calories per serving	10 calories per serving	50 calories	2,600 calories, or 0.75 pounds
Kraft Zesty Italian Salad Dressing, 109 calories per 2 Tbsp	Kraft 100% Fat Free Italian Salad Dressing, 20 calories per 2 Tbsp	89 calories per 2 Tbsp	445 calories	23,140 calories, or 6.6 pounds
Newman's Own Caesar Dressing, 150 calories per 2 Tbsp	Ken's Steak House Lite Caesar, 70 calories per 2 Tbsp	80 calories per 2 Tbsp	400 calories	20,800 calories, or about 6 pounds

THE POWER OF PREVENTION

Keeping a food journal does more than show you what you're eating—it also prompts you to *change* what you're eating. Just like Nicole, when you notice patterns that are undermining your weight-loss efforts, you'll be inspired to alter the way you eat.

Knowing that you have to hold yourself accountable for every morsel of food you eat also helps to keep you on track. When you walk by that person in the mall handing out free samples of fudge, you'll know that grabbing a chunk means you'll have to pull out your phone or food journal and make another entry. "One chunk of peanut butter fudge; 100+ calories." Just knowing you'll have to enter that information is motivation enough to keep walking.

The great thing about tracking your calories is that there will also be times when you'll be able to see clearly that you're on target to finish the day far from the Red Zone, meaning you have plenty of calories to spare. That's when you can take that sample of fudge without feeling guilty. And trust us, fudge tastes a lot better when you know it's not making you fat.

YES, YOU CAN (EAT WHAT YOU WANT)

That's right. You really can eat pizza (or burgers, or cupcakes, or whatever your "thing" is) and lose weight. As we've said before, it's all in the math. You can eat what you want and drop pounds just as long as you're burning more calories than you're consuming.

Of course, a million fad diets have insisted otherwise, telling us for years that you can't lose weight if you're eating carbs, fat, or whatever the dietary punching bag of the moment was. But at the end of the day, it doesn't matter if you choose to eat only carbs, fat, and sugar, or if you eat nothing but fiber and protein (though neither of these strategies is advisable, from a health perspective). If you come in under your calorie budget, you will lose weight.

Still skeptical? Well, ask the folks at Harvard for confirmation. In 2009, scientists at the Harvard School of Public Health published the results of a study in which they recruited 811 overweight people and randomly assigned them to follow one of four diets, each with different ratios of macronutrients, ranging from high-protein to low-carb to low-fat. The subjects were followed for 2 years—a period of time that is almost an eternity by the standards of most diet studies.

The results showed clearly that when it comes to weight loss, calories are king. When the subjects reduced the number of calories they consumed, they all lost weight, regardless of the breakdown of nutrients in their diets. Or, as the authors of the study stated it: "Reduced-calorie diets result in clinically meaningful weight loss regardless of which macronutrients they emphasize."

"The public might be confused as to what the perfect diet is, and this study suggests people should be focusing on counting calories," said one of the coauthors, Stephen D. Anton, a professor at the University of Florida who trained the dietitians that helped conduct the study.

"We've shown that any reasonable diet can provide weight loss, as long as caloric intake is reduced," said Katherine D. McManus, RD, MS, with the Department of Nutrition at Brigham and Women's Hospital in Boston. She coauthored the report, which was published in the *New England Journal of Medicine* and funded by the National Institutes of Health (NIH).

The message could not have been clearer: If you're trying to lose weight, then you *must* reduce calories.

TRACKING AND EYEBALLING

There's a reason that tracking your calories is the second pillar of the Lose It! philosophy: Once you start tracking, you'll learn exactly what you need to do to cut back on calories. Just like Nicole, who was shocked to discover that she was eating 3,000 calories a day (and that a large portion of those calories came from something as seemingly innocuous and healthy as skim milk) you are likely to be shocked when tracking reveals how much (and what) you've *really* been eating.

In fact, if you're like most Americans, then you've probably been eating two or three servings of food at every meal—or much, much more—without even knowing it. This is why many people have trouble understanding why they're not losing weight even when they're eating fairly healthy foods or only eating what they're served. In our super-sized environment, we've all been programmed to eat double or triple a normal portion size and think nothing of it.

According to the NIH, bagels made 20 years ago were 3 inches in diameter and only 140 calories, while a typical bagel today is double that size and has *more than* double the calories (350). Twenty years ago, two slices of pizza would've set you back 500 calories; today, they'll set you back at least 850. When McDonald's first opened its doors in 1955, its only hamburger weighed 1.6 ounces; now the largest patty tips the scales at 8 ounces, a whopping 500 percent growth. Even the Big Mac (540 calories) seems miniature in comparison to many of the chain's newer options. It's now outsized by at least four other burgers on the

McDonald's menu, including the Angus Deluxe (750 calories) and the Angus Bacon & Cheese (790 calories). The chart below offers more examples of the ever-expanding portion sizes being offered at many popular chain restaurants.

Stop the Supersizing Madness!

One Serving of	Has Roughly	But One Actual Order Has	If You Ate a Whole Order Once a Week for a Year It Would Equal
Pizza Hut's Tuscani Creamy Chicken Alfredo pasta	630 calories	2 servings, or 1,260 calories	65,520 calories, or 19 pounds
Pizza Hut's Pepperoni P'Zone Pizza	630 calories	2 servings, or 1,260 calories	65,520 calories, or 19 pounds
Domino's Pizza Buffalo Chicken Kickers	102 calories	5 servings, or 510 calories	26,520 calories, or 7.6 pounds
Domino's Pizza Cinna Stix	118 calories	8 servings, or 940 calories	48,880 calories, or 14 pounds
Domino's Pizza Grilled Chicken Caesar Salad with dressing and croutons	330 calories	2 servings, or 660 calories	34,320 calories, or 9.8 pounds
Papa John's Chickenstrips	130 calories	3.5 servings, or 455 calories	23,660 calories, or 6.8 pounds
Papa John's Applepie	480 calories	3 servings, or 1,440 calories	74,880 calories, or 21.4 pounds
Papa John's Garlic Parmesan Breadsticks	340 calories	5 servings, or 1,700 calories	88,400 calories, or 25.3 pounds

Recognizing and judging portion sizes is a crucial part of tracking your foods. If your hanger steak is literally hanging off your plate, then instead of eating about 300 calories—the amount in about 4 ounces, which is one serving—you'll be consuming double or triple that. If you're eating a healthy salad that's swimming in 6 tablespoons of ranch dressing (almost 500 calories), then guess what? You're not eating a salad with a serving of dressing, you're eating a bowl of ranch-flavored soup with chunks of vegetables.

So to ensure that you're keeping your eye on the prize, you must keep an eye on your portion sizes. Don't store your measuring cups in a drawer—keep them out on your kitchen counter where you can grab them in a pinch to measure portions of cereal, milk, pasta, and sauces. Kelly Akins Mayfield, a registered nurse in Alabama who's struggled with her weight for years, says that starting to measure her portion sizes at home was a huge wake-up call.

"Downloading Lose It! pretty much changed my life," she says. "I never realized how many calories I was eating. When I started tracking on Lose It!, I realized I was eating more than the serving size of many foods. If the serving size was 1 cup, for instance, I was often eating 3 cups. Even for cereal—a serving size is usually 1 cup or 1½ cups, and I was probably eating double or more. I was just overeating."

Kelly has been dropping pounds at a healthy pace for about a year, and she credits Lose It! and her new dedication to measuring portion sizes with helping her get on track.

"When I started using Lose It!, I was a little stubborn. But then, when I got into it, the weight just started dropping off. It was so easy. I'll probably use it for the rest of my life. When I start to feel like I've lost track of what I've been eating, it's so easy to pull out my phone and figure out how many calories I've eaten that day."

In addition to using measuring cups and spoons, some Lose It! users also keep a food scale on their counter. A food scale can come in handy when you're following a recipe (which may call for foods to be measured in ounces), but it's also helpful when determining the amount of food contained in a packaged product. Many food labels on packaged foods are pretty misleading, and food companies aren't always precise when it comes to the weights of their products. And because federal regulators are more likely to penalize a company for overstating the weight of a product or package of food than for understating it, some manufacturers will actually stuff more food in their packages than is indicated on the label. That can fool you into consuming many more calories than you think you are from foods like cookies, potato chips, crackers, and cereal. But weighing your food can help you avoid these covert calories. For instance, if the label on a box of crackers reads "net weight 14 ounces" and your food scale says the product weighs 16 ounces, you know there are some extra calories in the box, so it's important to record your calories.

Even if you're not going to weigh and measure all of your food all of the time, it's useful and educational to do it for your first few weeks. Doing this will give you a sense of what a portion should look like and will help to recalibrate your expectations of a serving size. After a while, you'll be able to eyeball your portions with accuracy. But keep in mind that when you introduce a new food that you're not used to eating—a new type of cereal, for instance—it's important to use the measuring cups again so you know exactly what a correct serving size looks like. Keep measuring each time until you know it by heart.

Measuring serving sizes in your own kitchen is one thing, but on someone else's turf, it can be trickier. On pages 46 and 47, you'll find a handy guide to serving sizes that will help you determine what's on your plate and how much of it you're eating.

1 ounce: One serving of cheese (one slice), as well as most snack foods, including nuts, chips, and pretzels

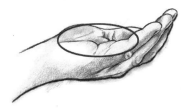

3 ounces: Approximately one serving of cooked fish, turkey, meat, or poultry

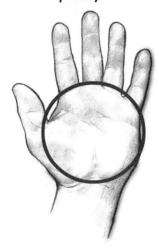

1 cup: Approximately one serving of cereal, soup, soda, cooked veggies, salad, milk, yogurt, casserole, stew, or chili

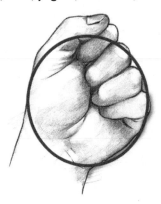

½ cup: One serving of ice cream, fruit or fruit juice, rice or noodles, beans, pasta, tomato sauce, or starchy vegetable (like potatoes and corn)

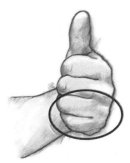

1 teaspoon: One serving of margarine, butter, oil, or mayo

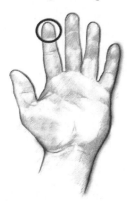

1 tablespoon: One serving of ketchup, salad dressing, jam, jelly, or cream cheese

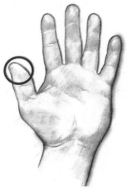

Illustrations courtesy of the National Institute of Diabetes and Digestive and Kidney Diseases

ARE ALL CALORIES CREATED EQUAL?

At the core of the Lose It! philosophy is the belief that you are your own expert. Decades of trendy diets have distorted the basic tenets of nutrition in an effort to justify extreme dieting. But that doesn't mean you should dismiss nutritional considerations from your weight-loss strategy. In fact, excluding any consideration of carbohydrates, protein, and fat from your food decisions is like drawing a square when what you want is a cube: It leaves out several dimensions. Calories represent the end goal, but taking in a little more protein and fiber along with the right carbs and fats will help you get the most bang for your calorie buck.

So in the interest of giving you the information you need to make better decisions, here's a quick rundown of the nutrients that will help keep you out of the Red Zone.

Foods That Help the Calorie Cause
Complex Carbs

Carbs are the favored punching bag of many diets these days. But complex carbs—the kind found in whole grains, fruits, and vegetables—help you lose weight in the long run. They're made of long molecules that your body has to work hard to metabolize, so you end up with a slow and steady source of energy and a blood sugar level that stays on a nice, even keel. That prevents those dreaded hunger-inducing insulin spikes that cause you to make a hard right every time your car approaches a Dairy Queen.

Your body needs carbs for fuel, and health officials say you should get between 45 and 65 percent of your daily calories from them. When you deprive yourself of this energy source, you force your body to dip into its carbohydrate reserves, which are stored in your liver and muscles in the form of glycogen molecules. Each molecule of glycogen is attached to several water molecules. That's why you lose weight so quickly on a carb-free diet—many of those initial lost pounds are nothing more than water weight. Unfortunately, it all comes right back as soon as you have so much as a breadstick.

Friendly Fats

Despite what we've all been told, eating a decent amount of fat can help you fend off flab much better than a low-fat diet can. In fact, humans have special fat receptors on our tongues that evolved to encourage us to seek out fat in times when food was scarce; this is because we need fat to produce hormones and facilitate proper body function. And all it takes is a bite of a cheeseburger to prove that fat is deliciously satiating; it has a pleasurable texture and mouthfeel that adds richness to our foods.

What's more, when you combine fat with simple carbs, the fat prevents spikes in blood sugar. One type of fat in particular, monounsaturated fat (found in olive oil, canola oil, nuts, and avocados), is a potent tummy trimmer. Monounsaturated fats enhance the body's breakdown of stored fat, and because they're the most satiating of all fats, they'll help you consume fewer calories. As a 2002 study in the *International Journal of Obesity* reported, people who were faced with the temptation of the bread basket at a restaurant ate 23 percent less bread when they used olive oil instead of butter as a condiment.

Health officials suggest that 20 to 35 percent of your daily calories should come from fat (all kinds).

Protein

Protein deserves a lot of praise. The building block of all human cells, it's also a veritable gut-be-gone that prevents weight gain by helping you feel

(continued on page 53)

THE TOP 10 FOODS THAT FILL YOU UP: THE CREAM OF THE CROP

As you search for ways to eat well and slim down, you'll want to lean toward foods that give you the highest serving of protein and fiber for the lowest calorie count. What we've gathered here, in no particular order, is a list of the top 10 foods that fit the bill—foods that'll fill you up without fattening you up.

1. **Fish.** Coldwater fish like salmon, mackerel, and tuna will give you plenty of protein and healthy fats without throwing too many calories your way. A 6-ounce fillet of salmon will deliver 34 grams of protein, plenty of healthy omega-3s, and only 4 grams of saturated fat for just 250 calories. A 6-ounce porterhouse, by comparison, would deliver 100 extra calories and four times the saturated fat for the same amount of protein.

2. **Quinoa**. One serving of this wonder grain—½ cup—has about 130 calories, 3 grams of fiber, and 6 grams of protein. You can find quinoa in any supermarket. Use it in place of white rice or add it to soups and oatmeal for a protein-and-fiber infusion.

3. **Nuts.** An ounce of peanuts has 166 calories, but plenty of heart-healthy fats to keep you full and satiated. Studies show that people who eat nuts lose more weight than those who don't, because nuts help control appetite. Keep packets of almonds, walnuts, or any other nuts (as long as they don't contain added sugars) at your desk or in your purse or gym bag for a quick snack. Or keep a jar of peanut butter in the fridge (look for all-natural varieties without added trans fats or hydrogenated oils) for a quick and cheap protein source.

4. **Lentils.** We know what you're thinking. How on earth am I going to eat lentils? But stick with us for a second. A cup of lentils (cooked) has only 230 calories but a stunning 18 grams of protein

and 16 grams of fiber. (That's 60 percent of your recommended daily fiber, based on a 2,000-calorie-a-day diet.) So here's how you use them: Think Hamburger Helper. When you're making burgers or meatballs, swap out some of the ground beef for mashed lentils. When you're cooking enchiladas, use lentils instead of rice or pinto beans. Making a bowl of chili? Throw in a quarter cup of cooked lentils. You'll never notice a difference.

5. **Greek yogurt.** Rich and creamy, hearty and filling, you can't go wrong with Greek yogurt. An 8-ounce serving of Fage Total 0% Greek yogurt has an almost invisible 120 calories but packs 20 grams of protein—and zero fat! Plus it has active cultures that aid digestive health and plenty of bone-strengthening calcium. Try it for breakfast, eat it as a sweet after-dinner treat with a little fruit or honey, or substitute it for sour cream in dips and other recipes.

6. **Avocados.** Don't be afraid of avocados. They get a bad rap for being high in fat, but most of that fat is monounsaturated. Half an avocado has 4 grams of protein and nearly 6 grams of fiber (the most of any fruit), but only 150 calories. That's less than the amount of calories in a small order of McDonald's french fries (230 calories); amazingly, it's even less than a single serving of most Caesar or blue cheese salad dressings (170 to 190 calories). When you want a hearty salad, top it with avocado slices and skip the salad dressing.

7. **Raspberries.** Nutritionists love berries for their disease-fighting antioxidants, and they get an A+ for their off-the-charts fiber content, as well. And at the head of the berry class is the mighty raspberry. One cup (a mere 50 calories) has 8 grams of belly-filling fiber. For most people, that's more than 25 percent of the recommended daily amount. Eat them fresh or buy them frozen—frozen berries are cheap, convenient, and have all the fiber and nutrients you'll find in fresh.

(continued)

THE TOP 10 FOODS THAT FILL YOU UP—*Continued*

8. **Whole wheat pasta.** Put your pasta to work for you. Americans love pasta with a passion, but unfortunately, the standard varieties are brimming with simple carbs and not much else. So make the switch to whole wheat. It costs and tastes about the same as white pasta, but it carries a blast of fiber and protein. One cup of whole wheat spaghetti (cooked) has 174 calories, 8 grams of protein, and almost 7 grams of fiber. Plus, unlike regular pasta, its complex carbs won't wreak havoc on your blood sugar and push your body into fat-storage mode.

9. **Broccoli.** It's hard to go wrong with any vegetable, but nothing packs more protein and fiber in a minuscule package of calories quite like broccoli does. One cup of cooked, chopped broccoli has barely 50 calories and a measly 11 grams of carbs (4 percent of the recommended daily amount, based on a 2,000-calorie-a-day diet). Yet somewhere in those 50 calories you'll find 4 grams of protein and more than 5 grams of fiber. That's a lot of bang for your buck.

10. **Oatmeal.** Nothing fills you up like a bowl of warm and hearty, stick-to-your-ribs oatmeal. It's one of the easiest ways to satisfy your stomach without super-sizing your waist. The reason? It's high in fiber, protein, and slow-to-digest complex carbs. A single cup of cooked oatmeal packs 6 grams of protein and 4 grams of fiber, all for only 166 calories. Forget Wheaties—oatmeal is the breakfast of champions (and a great snack, too). For best results, try making your oatmeal just like Mom used to: a pinch of salt, a little skim milk, and a drizzle of honey. Or add oats to your smoothies, cookies, soups, and ground beef or turkey for a blast of lean fiber.

full long after you've eaten, thereby reducing your appetite. But it also helps you slim down simply because higher-protein foods—such as lean meats, eggs, tofu, beans, grains, and some other plants—tend to have fewer calories than foods with more carbs and fat, which are generally more energy dense.

Health authorities recommend that between 10 and 35 percent of your calories should come from protein. But it's not a bad idea to err on the side of getting a little more, especially if you're exercising, since you'll need the extra protein to help build new muscle and repair the muscles you've been working.

Fiber

You can't go wrong with fiber. In fact, insoluble fiber—the kind found in whole grains, veggies, nuts, wheat, corn, bran, and some fruits—contains *zero* calories. Meanwhile, the other fiber—the soluble kind found in oats, beans, and fruits and veggies like carrots, oranges, and apples—regulates your blood sugar, preventing cravings and hunger pangs. And if you've ever chosen raisin bran over Froot Loops in the morning, you already know that fiber helps you feel full longer. The government recommends a *minimum* of 20 to 35 grams a day—women should be getting a minimum of 21 grams a day and men need at least 30. Yet most Americans consume roughly half of that amount, about 12 to 18 grams in a typical day. If you're not meeting your daily requirements, consider adding fiber to your morning meal. Breakfast is an especially good time to get in a dose of fiber because it helps you feel full, regulates blood sugar, and promotes digestive health. Many breakfast options—from whole-wheat toast to cereal, oatmeal, and fruit—provide a good dose. Boost your fiber intake and you'll boost your progress on the scale.

Foods That Hurt the Calorie Cause
Simple Carbs

Why are they called "simple"? Because they're just that—simple to metabo-lize. An influx of simple carbs from a bag of chips or cookies floods your bloodstream with sugar, which in turn triggers a flood of insulin. That signals your body to store some of the sugar as fat, and as soon as the sugar's all gone, you're hungry again. It's a belly-bloating cycle. This is not to say that you can't eat *any* simple carbs—life wouldn't be the same without the occasional Chips Ahoy! cookie. But replacing simple carbs with complex carbs from time to time will help you eat less food in the long run.

Trans Fats

Every health authority in America has railed against trans fats because they increase bad cholesterol (LDL) and reduce good cholesterol (HDL). And there's another good reason to keep an eye on them: They'll make you pack on pounds. A 2006 study by researchers at the Wake Forest Univer-sity School of Medicine showed that eating trans fats not only accelerates weight gain, it also makes fat more likely to gather around your waist. That's right—the dreaded belly fat. Trans fats are designed to extend the shelf life of foods, but they won't do anything to benefit *your* shelf life, or your waistline.

You don't have to make yourself crazy obsessing over carbs, protein, or fat. But it is a good idea to read food labels whenever possible and choose items that have more protein and fiber and fewer simple carbs. Why? Because if you feel full and satisfied, that leftover piece of cheesecake sitting in the fridge will hold a lot less power over you.

Paul Cassese of New York, 31, says he tried to give up carbs for years but was never able to do it. At 5 foot 9 and 215 pounds, he was about 40 pounds heavier than he wanted to be. Eventually, after his first child was born, Paul decided that he wanted to get serious about weight loss, so he gave Lose It! a shot.

"It takes determination to stick with it. But when all is said and done, I can't believe how easy losing weight is when you just break it down to a simple formula."

With the help of Lose It!, Paul now looks for foods that contain fewer calories but are more satisfying. Often that means making commonsense decisions to opt for foods that are high in fiber, protein, and complex carbs. In other words, he chooses the foods that give him the most satisfaction for the least amount of calories.

"When you start counting your calories, you really make better decisions. If I want ice cream and I'm really hungry, I know a serving is only ½ cup and that won't fill me up. So I'll eat something else instead that *will* satisfy me—even if that's a serving of chips. I've also started eating more healthy snacks and making better choices because I know what makes me feel full. My intake of fruits and vegetables has gone through the roof."

"I work in Manhattan," he notes, "And sometimes my lunch choices are limited to deli buffets. So I just make better choices in those situations. I've stopped going for the pasta and rice, and instead I fill up my plate with vegetables and lean proteins."

Paul still eats rice and pasta occasionally; he just eats less of these foods and makes sure his other choices keep him feeling full and satisfied. By following that strategy, Paul has reached his goal of losing 40 pounds, and he's been able to maintain that loss pretty easily.

"I have no plans to stop using Lose It!," he says. "It's become part of my lifestyle."

SMART SWAPS AT EVERY MEAL

Now that you're tracking your foods—and you've got an eye on portion sizes and the foods that'll help the cause, not hurt it—you're ready to make some smart swaps. Remember, your own personal weight-loss revolution takes place one meal at a time. The point isn't to give up the foods you love to eat, it's to look for ways to make those foods less costly from a calorie standpoint. That way, you can eat what you want and still lose weight. All you have to do is start implementing small, sustainable changes that you can stick with every day. Here are a few examples to help you get started. Consider it your cheat sheet to slimmer eats.

The Breakfast Club

If you walk out your door each morning without eating breakfast, you're missing out. Studies have consistently shown that people who skip breakfast are far more likely to be obese or overweight than those who do eat it. A light breakfast won't cost you many calories (a serving of cereal with ½ cup of skim milk is usually somewhere in the neighborhood of 200 calories), and because you've eaten something that stabilizes your blood sugar, you won't experience those midmorning hunger pangs that prompt you to reach for the nearest muffin. Eating breakfast also helps prevent you from going on a sugar or carb spree at lunchtime.

A 2002 study by the National Weight Control Registry found that 78 percent of people who maintained a weight loss of at least 30 pounds for 1 year—and some for as long as 6 years—ate breakfast every day. Having breakfast is like losing weight as you eat. It's an easy habit to get into, and it's a golden opportunity to make some smart swaps. As you can see from the chart below, making a few modifications to your daily cereal bowl can add up to a weight loss of almost 9 pounds over the course of a year!

Smarter Cereal Choices
(1 cup of each)

If Every Day You Swapped This	For This	Then You'd Save
Kellogg's Smart Start Original Antioxidants (190 calories)	General Mills Cheerios (100 calories)	2,520 calories a month, or almost 9 pounds a year
Kellogg's Raisin Bran (190 calories)	General Mills Fiber One Raisin Bran Clusters (170 calories)	560 calories a month, or 2 pounds a year
General Mills Apple Cinnamon Cheerios (160 calories)	Post Honeycomb (87 calories)	2,044 calories a month, or 7 pounds a year
General Mills Lucky Charms (147 calories)	Kellogg's Froot Loops (110 calories)	1,036 calories a month, or 3.5 pounds a year
Whole milk (150 calories)	Fat-free skim milk (90 calories)	1,680 calories a month, or 5.8 pounds a year
Rice Dream Heartwise Vanilla nondairy beverage (130 calories)	Almond Breeze Original nondairy beverage (60 calories)	1,960 calories a month, or 6.7 pounds a year

But cereal isn't the only breakfast item that's easy to overhaul. The chart on page 58 offers options for making more breakfast swaps that will save you hundreds—even thousands—of calories over the course of just a month.

Better Breakfast Breads, Bagels, and Meats

If Every Day You Swapped* This	For This	Then You'd Save
Wonder Bread, 2 slices (120 calories and 0 g of fiber)	Nature's Own Double Fiber Wheat bread, 2 slices (100 calories and 10 g of fiber)	560 calories a month, or 1.9 pounds a year
Thomas' New York Style Plain Bagel (290 calories and 3 g of fiber)	Thomas' Light Multi-Grain English Muffin (100 calories and 8 g of fiber)	5,320 calories a month, or 18.2 pounds a year
Kraft Philadelphia Cream Cheese, Original, 2 tablespoons (90 calories)	Kraft Philadelphia Whipped Cream Cheese, 2 table-spoons (60 calories)	840 calories a month, or 2.9 pounds a year
Smucker's Squeeze Grape Jelly, 1 tablespoon, (50 calories)	Welch's Reduced Sugar Concord Grape Jelly, 1 tablespoon (20 calories)	840 calories a month, or 2.9 pounds a year
Jimmy Dean Croissant Sandwich: Sausage, Egg, and Cheese (430 calories)	Jimmy Dean D-Lights Turkey Sausage Muffin (260 calories)	4,760 calories a month, or 16.3 pounds a year
Farmland Foods Hickory Smoked Bacon, 3 slices (120 calories)	Wellshire Farms Classic Sliced Turkey Bacon, 3 slices (60 calories)	1,680 calories a month, or 5.8 pounds a year

THE CALORIE CRUNCH AT LUNCH

Many Lose It! users find that lunch presents their biggest calorie pitfall of the day. It's typically your first large meal, and in the midst of a busy day it's easy to search for a little stress relief in a sandwich the size of a scud missile. But when you find yourself standing in line at a fast-food joint with a dizzying array of options, remember that you can always go big without *making* yourself big. All it takes is a few smarter decisions. For instance, let's say you typically go to Subway for lunch. It only takes a few easy swaps—like getting honey mustard instead of mayo, asking for two slices of cheese instead of four, or getting a Big Philly Cheesesteak instead of a Meatball Marinara—to stop yourself from packing on some serious pounds. Here are some more ideas.

A Sandwich Board Makeover

If 4 Times Each Week You Had	Each Time You Would Save	After 1 Week You Would Save	After 1 Month You Would Save	After 6 Months You Would Save	After 1 Year You Would Save
A 6" Turkey Breast sandwich with 2 slices of Cheddar instead of 4	60 calories	240 calories	960 calories, or 0.3 pounds	5,760 calories, or 1.6 pounds	11,520 calories, or 3.3 pounds
A 6" Subway Club with 1 serving of Fat Free Honey Mustard instead of mayo	80 calories	320 calories	1,280 calories, or 0.4 pounds	7,680 calories, or 2.2 pounds	15,360 calories, or 4.4 pounds
A 6" Subway Club with light mayo instead of regular mayo	60 calories	240 calories	960 calories, or 0.3 pounds	5,760 calories, or 1.6 pounds	11,520 calories, or 3.3 pounds
A 6" Turkey sandwich with 9-Grain Wheat Bread instead of Honey Oat Bread	50 calories	200 calories	800 calories, or 0.2 pounds	4,800 calories, or 1.4 pounds	9,600 calories, or 2.7 pounds
A 6" Big Philly Cheesesteak instead of a 6" Meatball Marinara sandwich	70 calories	280 calories	1,120 calories, or 0.3 pounds	6,720 calories, or 1.9 pounds	13,440 calories, or 3.8 pounds
A Footlong Oven Roasted Chicken sandwich instead of a Footlong Sweet Onion Chicken Teriyaki sandwich	85 calories	340 calories	1,360 calories, or 0.4 pounds	8,160 calories, or 2.3 pounds	16,320 calories, or 4.7 pounds
A Footlong Turkey Breast & Black Forest Ham sandwich instead of the Footlong Subway Club	43 calories	172 calories	688 calories, or 0.2 pounds	4,128 calories, or 1.2 pounds	8,256 calories, or 2.4 pounds

EVEN AT DINNER, YOU CAN MAKE YOURSELF THINNER

For many people who work all day and have little time to eat, dinner is the main meal of the day—and the heaviest. It's an occasion when you can easily eat a few too many forkfuls of shrimp scampi or find yourself swimming deep in a bowl of spaghetti Bolognese, dangerously close to the Red Zone. But you can make simple substitutions at dinner that will save you calories without leaving you hungry for more. The chart below offers some easy examples.

Thinner Dinner Swaps

If Every Day You Swapped This	For This	Then You'd Save
McDonald's Value Meal: Big Mac, large fries, and a large Coke (1,350 calories)	Big Mac, small fries, and a Diet Coke (770 calories)	16,240 calories a month, or 55.7 pounds a year
McDonald's Big Mac (540 calories)	McDonald's Double Cheeseburger (440 calories)	2,800 calories a month, or 9.6 pounds a year
McDonald's Premium Crispy Chicken Club Sandwich (630 calories)	Premium Grilled Chicken Classic Sandwich (420 calories)	5,880 calories a month, or 20.2 pounds a year
Bertolli Shrimp Scampi & Linguine, 1 serving (353 calories)	Birds Eye Shrimp Scampi, 1 serving (190 calories)	4,564 calories a month, or 15.6 pounds a year
Stouffer's Cheesy Tomato Rigatoni, 1 container (430 calories)	Amy's Bowls Stuffed Pasta Shells, 1 container (310 calories)	3,360 calories a month, or 11.5 pounds a year
Domino's Pizza 12" Cheese Pizza, 4 slices (440 calories)	Domino's Pizza 12" Veggie Pizza, 4 slices (400 calories)	1,120 calories a month, or 3.8 pounds a year
Domino's Pizza Buffalo Wings, 3 servings (660 calories)	Domino's Pizza Buffalo Chicken Kickers, 5 servings (510 calories)	4,200 calories a month, or 14.4 pounds a year
PF Chang's Beef with Broccoli on White Rice, 1 serving (440 calories)	PF Chang's Beef with Broccoli on Brown Rice, 1 serving (420 calories)	560 calories a month, or about 2 pounds a year
PF Chang's Crispy Honey Chicken on White Rice, 1 serving (680 calories)	PF Chang's Sesame Chicken on Brown Rice, 1 order (510 calories)	4,760 calories a month, or 16 pounds a year

TOMORROW IS ANOTHER DAY

In all journeys, there are setbacks and bumps in the road—and as anyone who has ever dieted knows, this is especially true when it comes to weight loss.

It's important to plan your meals in advance and try to brace yourself for binge-fest holidays like Thanksgiving and Christmas (or any holiday, for that matter) by upping your calorie burn or eating a little bit less in the days preceding the feast. But sometimes, despite your best efforts, you'll find yourself soaring into the Red Zone before you've even sat down to dinner or sampled a spoonful of that chocolate mousse you've been eyeing all night. At other times, life simply gets in the way: Chained to your desk until 3 p.m., you're tempted to eat leftover donuts for lunch; you visit relatives for the weekend and find yourself surrounded by a plethora of poor choices; you're trapped in a PTA meeting for hours with no sustenance on hand but an assortment of cookies and cupcakes.

The important thing is to keep your eye on the prize and not let these temporary slip-ups get you down. The key to success is patience and making consistent changes—changes that eventually become so routine that they turn into habits. When you think long term, you *will* see results. You just need to stick with your program long enough to see your changes pay off.

According to the national 2010 *Food & Health Survey,* nearly 40 percent of people trying to lose or maintain their weight say the most important factor that causes them to quit a diet is not seeing results quickly enough. Another 33 percent say they get discouraged when they simply feel they're not making enough progress. Let's say a week goes by, and in that week you manage to stay underbudget 5 days, but you end up stepping just over the line into the Red Zone the other 2 days. Guess what: At the end of the week, you'll still be in a good position because you stayed out of the red more often than not. In other words, you will *still* have lost weight. Maybe not the 2 pounds you were hoping for. But losing 1.5 pounds is better than losing nothing, and it's certainly better than gaining a pound.

If you keep up that strategy and stay in the Green Zone most days of the week, your patience will pay off. If you go overbudget, don't beat yourself up about it. One bad day is just that—it doesn't mean you're doomed to repeat the past. Everyone in the Lose It! community has had those days, and there's only one tried-and-true method of getting back on track: Go to bed, wake up in the morning, and start all over again. The next morning, you'll be back in the Green Zone.

That's the beauty of Lose It!—every day you start with a blank slate and a full calorie budget to spend as you see fit. (Imagine waking up each morning with a brand new wad of cash to spend by day's end!) You'll never be judged for the previous day's missteps; you know where you went wrong, and it's up to you to get back on track. The important thing is to learn from a setback—you only need to review your calorie log to see where the slipup occurred. And when you see where you went off track, you'll know how to avoid repeating that mistake the next time you're faced with a similar situation.

Chapter Three

Move It to Lose It

Unleash Your Inner Athlete

Now that you know how simple it is to lose weight by making small, commonsense changes to your diet and tracking the calories you consume, the next step is to start burning off some of those calories.

In this chapter, you'll learn to use exercise as a tool—a veritable secret weapon, actually—in your war on fat. You'll learn how to burn more calories in less time and get the absolute most out of your limited gym sessions, and you'll discover the simple, everyday movements and activities that will burn extra calories without even requiring you to break a sweat. Whether you're a beginner or a workout warrior, these tips and tricks—gleaned from hard data and the successful habits of Lose It! users—will help you maximize the belt-tightening benefits of exercise and create a buffer between you and the Red Zone. And best of all, you'll do it with a personalized activity plan that's tailored precisely to your needs, goals, interests, and fitness level.

MULTITASKING: COUNTING CALORIES WHILE YOU EXERCISE

Contrary to popular belief (and reality television), you don't need to spend 40 hours a week on a treadmill, huffing with fury until you collapse in a pool of sweat, in order to lose weight. And you don't need an angry, take-no-prisoners trainer barking orders at you to stay motivated, either.

Unless you're named Michael Phelps—and you have all day to do nothing but exercise, eat, sleep, and get massages—intense training just isn't sustainable for most people. So for those of us who aren't weight-loss reality stars or Olympic athletes, the best strategy is to make calorie reduction the core of our weight-loss plan and to choose activities that will burn the greatest number of calories in the shortest amount of time. With Lose It!, efficiency and the calorie count are the name of the game.

WHAT HAS EXERCISE DONE FOR YOU LATELY?

So what exactly will exercise do for you?

For starters, exercise (any kind of exercise) will help you scale the weight-loss mountain faster than reducing your calorie intake alone will. It will also help you keep off the weight over the long haul. Researchers at the Harvard School of Public Health confirmed this in 2009 when they pooled and analyzed data from 18 different studies that examined what happened when overweight people either combined diet and exercise or just dieted alone. The results of this megastudy were clear: "Diet-plus-exercise interventions provided significantly greater weight loss than diet-only interventions."

Another group of researchers at Rio de Janeiro State University in Brazil quantified this difference. Their findings, published in the *International*

Journal of Obesity in 2005, revealed that people who combined diet and exercise lost an average of 28.6 pounds, compared to 21.8 pounds among people who dieted alone. Perhaps more significantly, the exercisers continued to outpace the couch potatoes; after a year, those who exercised maintained a 20 percent greater "sustained" weight loss.

Twenty percent may not sound like a lot, but it's pretty significant. It's the difference between losing 30 pounds and 36 pounds, or between losing 40 pounds and 48 pounds. Think about it in financial terms: If your boss told you he'd raise your annual salary by 20 percent if you worked an extra 3 hours over the course of each week, would you do it?

Of course you would. How could anyone say no? Twenty percent is the difference between $50,000 and $60,000, or $100,000 and $120,000. For most people, that's an offer that can't be refused. So if you wouldn't turn down 20 percent more money, then why would you turn down 20 percent more weight loss when the cost is only a few hours a week of getting physical? (Or less, as you're about to see.)

For Kevin K. Johnson, a busy supervisor at a cable company in Michigan and the father of two small children, a combination of exercise and calorie tracking resulted in significant weight loss. Kevin knew he was in trouble when he surpassed the limits of his digital bathroom scale. He was used to seeing a number somewhere around 330 pounds when he weighed himself. Then one day he stepped on the scale and saw nothing but error messages.

"That was a wake-up call," he says.

Kevin soon found Lose It! and almost immediately did two things. First, he changed his eating habits, on some days preparing food and bringing it to work and on others using Lose It! to look up foods and their calorie counts before he got to local restaurants so he'd know what to order. And second, he signed up to run a local 5K several months in

(continued on page 68)

CHOOSE YOUR REWARDS WHEN YOU BURN MORE CALORIES

The Centers for Disease Control and Prevention (CDC) recommends at least 2½ hours of moderate-intensity aerobic activity each week. If you exercise moderately for 3 hours each week in addition to tracking your calories and sticking within the limits of your budget, you can use exercise as a way to treat yourself to a few extra calories.

This is not to suggest that you should follow every trip to the gym with a burger and fries. The point is that exercise provides a little breathing room in your calorie budget and an opportunity to reward yourself with a favorite treat now and then.

Here's an idea of how you could reward yourself for 3 hours of cardio each week.

If Every Week You Did 3 Hours of	You Would Burn	Over the Course of 6 Months You Would Lose	Or Every Week You Could Treat Yourself to the Equivalent of
Aerobics			
155-pound person	1,256 calories	9.3 pounds	6 Original Glazed Krispy Kreme Donuts
200-pound person	1,620 calories	12 pounds	2 Sonic Jr. Double Cheeseburgers and Sonic Vanilla Shake
Bicycling			
155-pound person	1,367 calories	10.2 pounds	2 Applebee's Quesadilla Burgers and a Mesquite Chicken Salad
200-pound person	1,764 calories	13.1 pounds	3 McDonald's Quarter Pounders with Cheese and Hamburger
Dance Classes			
155-pound person	1,060 calories	7.9 pounds	4 scoops of Baskin-Robbins Oreo Cookies 'n Cream Ice Cream
200-pound person	1,368 calories	10.2 pounds	Half slab of ribs and slice of Junior's cheesecake

If Every Week You Did 3 Hours of	You Would Burn	Over the Course of 6 Months You Would Lose	Or Every Week You Could Treat Yourself to the Equivalent of
Jogging 155-pound person	2,092 calories	15.5 pounds	Slice of red velvet cake, Philly cheesesteak sandwich, and Pepperidge Farm chicken potpie
200-pound person	2,700 calories	20 pounds	5 Nestlé Toll House chocolate chip cookies, 4 Oreo cookies, and 2 slices of Amy's Kitchen Cheese Lasagna
Spinning 155-pound person	1,479 calories	11 pounds	Medium bag of AMC movie popcorn, large Coke, box of Milk Duds, and 5th Avenue candy bar
200-pound person	1,908 calories	14.2 pounds	2 Boston Market Chocolate Chip Fudge Brownies, side of Macaroni and Cheese, and Triple Topped Chicken dish
Stair Climbing 155-pound person	1,897 calories	14.1 pounds	Entire pint of Häagen-Dazs Vanilla ice cream and 4 slices of Pizza Hut thin crust cheese pizza
200-pound person	2,448 calories	18.2 pounds	Burger King Steakhouse XT Value Meal (with small Coke and fries), 2 slices of Hershey's Sundae Pie, and small Chocolate Shake
Brisk Walking 155-pound person	1,228 calories	9.1 pounds	4 Godiva chocolate truffles and large (8 oz) sirloin steak
200-pound person	1,584 calories	11.8 pounds	Baskin-Robbins Chocolate Chip Cookie Dough Sundae and 2 regular-size cones with Vanilla Soft Serve ice cream
Yoga 155-pound person	1,116 calories	8.3 pounds	2 Big Macs
200-pound person	1,440 calories	10.7 pounds	McDonald's McRib sandwich, large order of fries, and regular-size Chocolate Triple Thick Shake

advance, which inspired him to exercise for about 30 minutes most days to get in shape.

"I used it as additional motivation to work out," he says. "I would ride a bike or run. At my local gym, I would run in the pool and just focus on keeping my arms under the water, and just going back and forth for half an hour. Just this last week I bumped it up to 40 minutes."

Within a year, Kevin had lost 85 pounds. He was also happier than ever.

"I'm loving it. Keeping track of my exercise helps motivate me to keep track of my calories—I can see how each element influences the other. You can't really have one without the other. I need both of them to keep track of everything—calories in and calories out. And it's nice to see when I've eaten all my calories for the day and I've worked out that I've burned an additional 700 calories. It's kind of cool to see my progress."

MORE CALORIES OUT MEANS MORE CALORIES IN

We know that exercise helps us to lose weight faster—a pretty powerful motivator to get moving. But exercise offers other health benefits as well, such as lower blood pressure, better cardiovascular health, and decreased risk for many diseases. It also provides a few enticing incentives that make the weight-loss journey a bit more pleasant. In fact, for many Lose It! users, one of the biggest motivations to exercise is the opportunity to add *more calories to their daily budget.* Exercise can help you stay in the Green Zone even when you make the "wrong" choice (see the chart on the opposite page) or splurge on a favorite high-calorie food. That means that if you're going out to dinner and you know you'll need a couple hundred extra calories in your budget, a trip to the gym can buy you the extra calories you need in the form of sweat equity.

HOW TO *REWIND* THE CALORIE CLOCK

It's 4 o'clock. You're hungry. It's decision time: You could either make the "right" choice and have an energy bar, or you could go for what you *really* want and eat a Snickers bar, instead. You go for the Snickers bar. Later, you're feeling guilty about the splurge. But guess what? From a caloric standpoint, you can magically turn that Snickers bar into an energy bar. All it takes is the right amount of exercise to rewind the clock and make up the calorie difference between the "right" choice and *your* choice!

Here are a few ways you can turn back the calorie clock on an indulgent snack.

If You Went with This (the "Bad" Choice)	Instead of This (the "Right" Choice)	The Difference Would Be	But You Could Rewind the Calorie Clock with
Starbucks Blueberry Scone (460 calories)	Starbucks Dark Cherry Yogurt Parfait (310 calories)	150 calories	20 minutes on the elliptical at moderate intensity (170 calories burned)
Snickers bar (280 calories)	Kashi GOLEAN Roll! bar, Chocolate Peanut (190 calories)	90 calories	10 minutes on the StairMaster at moderate intensity (90 calories burned)
Lay's Classic potato chips, 1 bag (150 calories)	Red Delicious apple (80 calories)	70 calories	15 minutes on the stationary bike at light intensity (80 calories burned)
McDonald's Strawberry Triple Thick Shake, 16 oz (560 calories)	Jamba Juice Banana Berry Smoothie, 16 oz (270 calories)	290 calories	30 minutes of jogging, or about 2.5 miles (295 calories burned)
Peanut M&M'S, 1 bag (250 calories)	Planters Trail Mix, Fruit & Nut, 1 serving (140 calories)	110 calories	10 minutes of jumping rope at moderate intensity (110 calories burned)

*All information in this chart is based on a 160-pound person.

Lose It! users are living proof that this strategy works. Take 50-year-old Alain Ponze of Florida, who has been able to lose more than 40 pounds with Lose It! Alain manages a French restaurant outside of Miami; the most fattening, calorie-rich dishes are always at his fingertips.

"Every time I go into the kitchen, there's something left over—a little foie gras, a little of this, a little of that. And I'm French, so I love to eat. I love meat, I love bread, I love cheese."

Alain began implementing small diet and lifestyle changes that have added up to big weight loss. He still eats delicious food that satisfies his French palate, but he's made some smart swaps from high-calorie items to lower-calorie substitutions. For instance, he switched from rich, calorie-dense Brie cheese to much-lower-calorie feta and mozzarella; replaced his crusty baguettes with lighter alternatives like pita and whole wheat bread; swapped out some (but not all) of the red meat in his diet in favor of chicken and fish; and started using more herbs, olive oil, and spices in his dishes, instead of sticking to heavy, butter- and cream-based sauces.

But when Alain still found himself craving sweets and snacks or needing more room in his calorie budget, he turned to his secret weapon: exercise. Alain began to take fast walks or jogs with his girlfriend and was able to add several hundred calories to his budget in just 30 or 40 minutes. Over time, Alain's walks and jogs have gradually turned into long-distance runs—and he's burning more calories than ever before. He now runs anywhere from 20 to 30 miles a week. It's a sharp reversal for a man who once hated running and just 8 months earlier didn't have the stamina to jog even half a mile.

"I firmly believe that 75 percent of losing weight is on your plate, and

SWAPPING IN FLAVOR, SWAPPING OUT FAT (BODY FAT, THAT IS)

With a Frenchman's hard-to-please palate and a chef's high standards, Alain Ponze loves a good, hearty meal. But to lose the weight, he combined exercise with a smattering of smart swaps, like trading red meat for chicken, fish, and eggs. Here's a look at a few of his swaps and how many calories they help him save.

The Old	The New	The Difference	Swap the Old for the New 5 Times a Week for a Year and You'll Save
Brie cheese, 75 g or roughly ½ cup (250 calories)	Mozzarella, part-skim, 75 g (190 calories)	60 calories	15,600 calories, or about 4.5 pounds
	Feta cheese, 75 g, (198 calories)	52 calories	13,520 calories, or about 3.9 pounds
Baguette, 6" (185 calories)	Pita (80 calories)	105 calories	27,300 calories, or about 7.8 pounds
	Whole wheat bread, 2 slices (100 calories)	85 calories	22,100 calories, or about 6.3 pounds
Beef, rib eye, 4 oz (308 calories)	Chicken breast, 4 oz (136 calories)	172 calories	44,720 calories, or about 12.8 pounds
	Sardines, 1 can or 2.6 oz (120 calories)	188 calories	48,880 calories, or about 14 pounds
Beef, skirt steak, 4 oz (228 calories)	Branzino (fish), 4 oz (110 calories)	118 calories	30,680 calories, or about 8.8 pounds
	Egg, hard-boiled (78 calories)	150 calories	39,000 calories, or about 11 pounds

the rest is exercise," he says. "It's a combination of cutting calories, eating good food, and getting exercise."

Alain's transformation has taken place inside and out. As he lost weight, his overall health improved. His cholesterol plummeted 63 points, from 230 to 167, and his waist size dropped from a 38 to a 32.

"Last week I went for a checkup, and the nurse was impressed when she saw the color of my blood—it was like pinot noir," he says. "If you don't exercise, your blood is a dark red color. The more you exercise, the more oxygen there is in your blood, so it's a lighter color. So just by the color, she could say to me, 'You're in good shape.'"

In Alain's story, there's an important theme: He was motivated by *food.* Most exercise programs miss the fact that real people, ordinary Americans just like you, enjoy eating. As Alain's story demonstrates, there's nothing wrong with liking calorie-rich foods. As long as you stay within your budget—and use exercise to build in a little wiggle room—you can eat the foods you love and still lose weight.

BURN CALORIES IN YOUR SLEEP

Weight loss, as you know, boils down to simple arithmetic. You'll never lose a single pound if at the end of the day you're still taking in as many calories as you're burning. When you don't create a calorie deficit, you don't lose weight.

Exercise not only gives you the immediate benefit of padding your calorie budget with a little extra space, it also offers long-term benefits that supplement your weight-loss efforts. Physical activity raises your metabolism (the rate at which you burn calories) so that your body keeps burning

Need to Burn Off Dessert?

Ate This?	Do This!	A 160-Pound Person Will Burn	a 200-Pound Person Will Burn	a 240-Pound Person Will Burn
Famous Amos Chocolate Chip cookies, 1 pack (280 calories)	30 minutes of aerobics, high impact	255 calories	319 calories	382 calories
Chips Ahoy! Chewy cookies, 3 (200 calories)	30 minutes of aerobics, low impact	183 calories	228 calories	273 calories
Oreo cookies, 3 (160 calories)	30 minutes of biking at a leisurely pace	146 calories	182 calories	218 calories
Dannon Light & Fit Peach yogurt, 1 container (80 calories)	30 minutes of walking at 2 mph	91 calories	114 calories	137 calories
Häagen-Dazs Chocolate Peanut Butter ice cream, ½ cup (360 calories)	30 minutes of jogging at 5 mph	292 calories	364 calories	436 calories
Pepperidge Farm Milk Chocolate Chunk Macadamia Nut Cookies, 4 (560 calories)	30 minutes of jogging at 8 mph	493 calories	615 calories	736 calories
Skinny Cow Low Fat Ice Cream Sandwich, Vanilla (140 calories)	About 30 minutes of bowling	110 calories	137 calories	164 calories
Klondike Original ice cream bar (250 calories)	60 minutes of weightlifting, free weights or machines	220 calories	274 calories	328 calories

calories at a higher rate long after you leave the gym. Scientists call this the "afterburn" effect. Regular exercise (especially strength training) also increases your body's percentage of lean muscle mass. Muscle is more metabolically active than fat, so the more of it you have, the more calories you burn, even at rest. That's right—exercise truly helps you burn calories as you sleep!

THE CALORIE CRUNCH: MAXIMIZE YOUR TIME

Think you don't have enough time to exercise? Think again. You're about to meet a number of Lose It! users—from a workaholic programmer to a nurse who works 12-hour shifts—who are just as busy as you are. If they can find the time to squeeze in a few quick workouts every week, so can you.

Because your time is limited, you probably want your workout to give you as much benefit as possible in the shortest time possible, and the absolute best way many Lose It! users do that is to supercharge their workouts with interval training: alternating short bursts of high-intensity work with easy-does-it recovery periods. A standard interval workout takes no more than 30 minutes and will benefit you in a multitude of ways. With these workouts, you'll save time and you'll burn more fat and calories than you would if you spent 30 minutes exercising at a moderate intensity level.

Short Bursts, Huge Gains

Interval training was originally designed for Olympic athletes, who can handle strenuous workouts. But in recent years, research on a range of people, including the elderly, has shown that people of all fitness levels can benefit from interval sessions when they're done a couple times a week. In fact, interval training has been shown to be several times more effective than old-fashioned exercise.

A study published in the *Journal of Physiology* in 2010 showed that doing ten 1-minute sprints on a standard stationary bike with about 1 minute of rest in between each burst on 6 days during a 2-week period was the equivalent—in terms of calories burned and stamina gained—of doing 10 hours of moderate bicycling in the same time period. In other words, doing six 20-minute exercise sessions every other day—a mere 2 hours in 2 weeks—offered the same benefits as 10 hours of exercise performed at a more moderate pace. And these subjects weren't professional athletes in peak condition—they were regular people who bicycled at a level of intensity that was very challenging, but still only half of what they could do at an all-out pace.

But you don't have to make interval training the focus of all of your workouts. In fact, a study published in the *Journal of Applied Physiology* in 2007 showed that after some initial interval training—alternating sets of 4 minutes of hard bike-riding with 2 minutes of rest—subjects burned 36 percent more fat on subsequent days when they switched to an hour of moderate cycling. They also boosted their cardiovascular fitness by 13 percent. Whether they were fit or sedentary before the study made no difference—in the end, they all improved their fat-burning capacity by comparable amounts. The conclusion is clear: Even if you incorporate interval training into your exercise routine only once or twice a week, you will reap the calorie-burning rewards.

Pretty much any type of cardiovascular exercise can be done in intervals: swimming, biking, jogging, walking, stair-climbing, even using the elliptical machine. The only difference is that instead of keeping up your usual steady pace while performing these exercises, you mix things up with bursts of speed and intensity.

But before you try this—or any of the exercises suggested in this book—make sure you're physically capable of the challenge. If you have heart disease, high blood pressure, arthritis, diabetes, or any other health issues that might pose a problem, check with your doctor before getting started. But if the only thing holding you back is a few extra pounds and a fear of pushing yourself too hard, it's time to get out of your comfort zone and get into the gym with one of the interval programs listed on the following pages.

TWO INTERVAL PROGRAMS TO TRY

Interval Program 1

This standard interval program involves three basic steps. You can do these with almost *any* cardio exercise, including swimming, running, stair-climbing, biking, and jogging on the treadmill.

When you're doing intervals, you don't need a wristwatch to figure out when to sprint and when to rest; your iPod or iPhone will do it for you. Go to cardiocoach.com and download one of their popular audio workouts. The site has MP3s for 20-minute intervals that'll let you know when to speed up and when to slow down.

Most cardio machines at your gym have interval settings as well, so the machines will speed up and slow down at just the right times.

AFTERBURN: THE GIFT THAT KEEPS ON SLIMMING

Remember, every time you step out of the gym or unlace your sneakers after a run, your body goes into afterburn mode and continues to torch calories. Exercise afterburn is influenced by several factors—gender, body size, the length of your workout, and so on—but one of the most important factors is the *intensity* of your workout (see page 84). The greater the intensity, the greater the postexercise burn. Here's a look at some of the greatest afterburners. Remember, these calories are in addition to what you burn while actually working out.

If You	You'd Have an After-Burn of Roughly	If You Did It 4 Days a Week, That Would Equal	So in 1 Year You'd Lose
Walked on a treadmill at 70% of your VO2 max* for 20 minutes	43 calories	172 calories	2.6 pounds
Walked on a treadmill at 70% of your VO2 max* for 40 minutes	49 calories	196 calories	3.0 pounds
Walked on the treadmill at 70% of your VO2 max* for 60 minutes	76 calories	304 calories	4.5 pounds
Jogged at 70% of your VO2 max* for 30 minutes	34.5 calories	138 calories	2.0 pounds
Ran intervals: 20 bouts of 1-minute duration at maximum effort	75 calories	300 calories	4.5 pounds
Circuit trained for 40 minutes, doing 15 reps per set at 50% of your 1-rep max**	50 calories	200 calories	3.0 pounds
Did 40 minutes of heavy resistance lifting, doing 3 to 8 reps per set at 80% of your 1-rep max**	51 calories	204 calories	3.0 pounds

*VO2 max, or maximal oxygen uptake, refers to the maximum amount of oxygen that your body can use during intense exercise.
** The most weight you can lift for one repetition with good form
Note: The numbers in this chart are averages and will vary slightly among individuals.

1: Begin with 3 to 5 minutes of warm-up (start out very light, at low intensity, and gradually increase the intensity at the end of the warm-up period). If you're on the treadmill, for example, start at a low speed and gradually increase to a moderate speed as you warm up. If you're swimming, start out with 3 to 5 minutes of laps at a slow and easy pace, gradually increasing the pace until you're swimming at a moderate speed.

2: Perform 1 minute of moderate- or high-intensity work followed by 1 minute of low-intensity work; repeat 6 to 8 times. If you're jogging outside or on the treadmill, that would mean sprinting at 80 percent effort or more for 1 minute (see the explanation of perceived effort on page 84), then slowing down to a gentle pace for the second minute, and repeating the cycle 6 to 8 times. If you're on a bike, it means getting up out of the saddle for a minute and going as hard as you can before slowing down for a second minute and then repeating the cycle 6 to 8 times.

3: End with 3 to 5 minutes of cooldown (light, low-intensity work that you gradually decrease by the end of the cooldown period). Okay, you've done 6 to 8 intervals and maxed out. This is where you slow down and ease your way out of the exercise. If you're in a pool, you glide through a few more laps. If you're on the treadmill and had the machine set at a speed of 7 to 10, this is where you bring it down to half that speed or even a little less, gradually decreasing it until you're walking. After the intervals, you should be exhausted.

Interval Program 2

Here's a variation on the standard routine. It starts off with shorter bursts that pyramid up and then gradually shrink down again. Just like the previous routine, the beauty of it is that it can be applied to almost any cardio routine—swimming, running, biking, walking, you name it.

1. 3 to 5 minutes of warm-up

2. 30 seconds of high-intensity work, followed by 1 minute of low-intensity work

3. 45 seconds of high-intensity work, followed by 1 minute of low-intensity work

4. 60 seconds of high-intensity work, followed by 1 minute of low-intensity work

5. 90 seconds of high-intensity work, followed by 1 minute of low-intensity work

6. 60 seconds of high-intensity work, followed by 1 minute of low-intensity work

7. 45 seconds of high-intensity work, followed by 1 minute of low-intensity work

8. 30 seconds of high-intensity work, followed by 1 minute of low-intensity work

9. 3 to 5 minutes of cooldown

STRENGTH TRAINING 101: BUSTING MYTHS ABOUT HEAVY LIFTING

You see it in the gym every day: People doing endless reps of very light weights, seemingly exerting little effort. Ask them why, and they'll tell you that they don't want to "bulk up" by lifting heavier weights—that doing more repetitions of lighter weights will produce better tone and definition.

It's hard to say how this bit of misinformation became so popular, but it's wrong, wrong, wrong. The research is in, and it very clearly shows that the best way to burn the most calories and achieve killer definition is to apply the same concept to strength training that you do to your cardio: The more intense and efficient, the better. That means lifting heavier weights—or more specifically, "challenging" weights—for fewer reps.

In a 2002 study, researchers looked at what happened when women performed various resistance exercises at different weights and repetitions (85 percent of their maximum ability for 8 reps, versus 45 percent for 15 reps). The women who did fewer reps with heavier weights burned more calories and had a greater metabolic boost after they exercised than those who did more reps with lighter weights.

Don't worry—just because you're lifting heavier weights doesn't mean you're going to end up looking like Hulk Hogan. Creating bulky, body builder–style muscles requires not only frequent heavy-lifting sessions but also heavy calorie consumption. Since you're already on a plan to reduce

TAKE A SPIN THROUGH THE STORE— THE APP STORE!

If you have an iPod or iPhone, download iTunes and go to the app store for an array of health and fitness–related apps. Here are a few recommendations to get you started.

RunKeeper, Free

There's a reason RunKeeper is one of the most popular exercise downloads in the app store. RunKeeper uses the iPhone 3G's built-in GPS to track your runs like a hawk. It records distance, duration, speed, pace, rise, and altitude, and it shows you a map detailing your run. But it's not just for runs. You can keep track of hikes, walks, bike rides, and ski runs and your workout information is uploaded to runkeeper.com, where you can view your progress.

iFitness, $1.99

Like a personal trainer on your iPhone, this app provides detailed instructions for a range of exercises and allows you to create your own your calorie intake, you'll end up evaporating body fat and replacing it with lean muscle, which will put you on the path toward reaching a physique that anyone would envy.

For most weightlifting exercises, you should use a weight that's heavy enough that you can only complete 8 to 12 reps with proper form (2 to 4 sets are ideal, with 1 to 2 minutes of rest between sets). You should be able to finish the last rep of each set with difficulty, but without breaking your form. With that strategy, you'll boost your metabolism, challenge your muscles enough to stimulate growth, and burn body fat.

In fact, strength training two or three times a week with *challenging*

custom workouts. You can even log your exercise according to specific body parts or muscle groups. Beginners will find the pointers and instructions especially useful.

Men's Health Workouts or *Women's Health* Workouts, $1.99 each

If you're a fan of the most comprehensive health and fitness magazines around, then take 'em with you to the gym. The apps track your reps and sets; allow you to e-mail your results to yourself or someone else; and provide unique workouts designed by top strength coaches, athletes, and fitness experts (along with easy-to-follow instructions and high-quality pictures). Plus, you'll find cool little tips and tricks.

Runner's World SmartCoach, $1.99

Fill out a few quick questions, provide a couple of details, and SmartCoach whips up a unique training plan that takes into account your current fitness level and shows you the best way to reach your goal. When you're ready for your workout, just pull up the app and it'll show you your plan for the day.

(but not overly heavy) weights is a strong predictor of lasting weight loss and, in particular, reduced body fat. A 2009 study conducted by researchers at the University of Arizona tracked 122 women for 6 years as they completed various amounts of exercise. The women who ultimately lost the most weight and body fat were those who did resistance exercises three times a week, performing sets of 8 reps at 70 to 80 percent of their ability. (To learn more about perceived exertion, see page 84.)

Sean Willson, a computer programmer in Illinois, is living proof of the amazing results that tracking calories and a little strength training can produce together. Sean, a busy father with two small children, has lost more than 100 pounds with Lose It! When Sean began the program, he carried 390 pounds on his 6-foot-2 frame, a result of poor eating habits mostly encouraged by his sedentary, workaholic lifestyle.

"I had the perfect job to not eat right. I sat in front of the computer all day, drinking soda and ordering pizza."

But tracking his food intake opened his eyes to exactly how much he was eating and made him decide that he had to hold himself accountable for his deteriorating health. Sean began by making some important improvements in his diet, cutting back on junk and processed food, cooking and barbecuing more often at home instead of eating out, and being more careful about his portion sizes. His next big step was implementing a workout plan that would maximize his calorie burn, which he accomplished by doing high-intensity circuit training several days a week. The circuit workouts are a mixture of cardio and weight training—and he does it all right in the basement of his own home with a few free weights, a workout DVD, and some cheap mats that he throws on the floor. In a circuit workout, you're basically performing 1 set of 10

(continued on page 96)

GIRL, YOU GOT TO CARRY THAT WEIGHT!

In a 2007 University of Pennsylvania study, a group of overweight and obese women between the ages of 25 and 44 was instructed to strength train with challenging weights twice a week, while another group was given brochures recommending aerobic exercise. Here's what happened after 2 years.

	At Baseline	Change After 2 Years
Body Fat		
Strength Training Group	44.3 percent	−3.68 percent
Aerobics Group	43.5 percent	−0.14 percent
Fat Mass		
Strength Training Group	76.6 pounds	−1.61 percent
Aerobics Group	74 pounds	+2.87 percent
Lean Mass		
Strength Training Group	95.6 pounds	+4.17 percent
Aerobics Group	95.5 pounds	+2.82 percent
Intraabdominal Fat		
Strength Training Group	71.8 cm^2	7 percent
Aerobics Group	67.4 cm^2	21 percent
Subcutaneous Abdominal Fat		
Strength Training Group	269 cm^2	0.97 percent
Aerobics Group	252 cm^2	6.12 percent

Source: *American Journal of Clinical Nutrition*
Source: *The Harvard Heart Letter*, July 2004, September 2007

PERCEIVED EXERTION:
HOW HARD ARE YOU WORKING OUT?

Sometimes it seems like any time spent at the gym is exhausting, but the truth is, there are variations in your level of intensity depending on the activity you're doing and how much effort you're putting in. The simplest rule of thumb, the "talk test," comes from the CDC. If you're doing a moderate-intensity activity, you'll be able to talk, but not sing, as you chug along. If you step it up to the point where you can say no more than a few words without stopping for a breath, then you're doing vigorous activity.

For a more precise measurement, scientists developed something called the Borg Scale, which allows you to monitor yourself using a scale of 6 to 20. Because the scale has a wide range, it takes using it a few times to get used to the number assessments, but you'll find that it works pretty well. Just try to judge your level of exertion honestly, thinking only about your overall level of intensity without focusing specifically on one ache or pain or on single body parts like your legs or arms. Think about your total level of effort, fatigue, and physical stress. How strenuous is this exercise?

Moderate intensity activities include the following:

> Biking under 10 miles per hour

> Tennis (doubles)

> Walking briskly at 3 miles per hour or faster

> Water aerobics

> Light gardening

Vigorous intensity activities include the following:

> Biking over 10 miles an hour

> Race walking, jogging, or running

> Tennis (singles)

> Swimming laps

> Jumping rope

> Heavy gardening

Borg Scale

6. 20 percent effort

7. Extremely light.

8. 40 percent effort

9. Very light. For a healthy person, this is easy walking at your own pace.

10. 55 percent effort

11. Light.

12. 65 percent effort

13. Somewhat hard. It's challenging, but you feel okay to continue.

14. 75 percent effort

15. Hard.

16. 85 percent effort

17. Very hard; strenuous. You can still go on, but you have to push yourself. You feel fatigued.

18. About 90 percent effort

19. Extremely hard and strenuous. For most people, this is the most difficult exercise they've ever experienced.

20. Maximal exertion.

BANISH FAT AND BUILD MUSCLE

Short-Circuit Your Belly Fat with This Strength Training Routine

The purpose of circuit training is to keep your body by moving from one set of the exercises to the next with little or no rest in between, hitting every major muscle group along the way. The beauty of circuit training is that your routine is never set in stone: You can mix and match your exercises, as long as you knock out 10 different exercises that hit every major muscle group. You should try to do at least two circuits per session, giving yourself a minimum of 2 minutes of rest between each circuit.

These exercises were culled from the successful routines of Lose It! users like Sean and combined with circuit-training suggestions from the CDC. For every exercise, you should use a weight that's comfortable but challenging. Choose one that will allow you to do 8 to 12 reps with proper form, which, according to various studies, will deliver the best fat- and calorie-burn. Perform this workout 2 or 3 days a week, using alternate days for cardio workouts (at least one of which should be intervals!).

PUSH-UPS

This exercise is the king of upper-body strengtheners. It works your chest, shoulders, arms, back, and core. But you must maintain proper form. To start, place your hands on the ground, keeping your back and legs straight as a board. Hands should be about shoulder-width apart. Push up and pause for a moment at the top. Slowly lower yourself to your starting position, making sure not to drop yourself too quickly. (The difficulty of the lowering movement, when done slowly, is where you pick up gains in strength.) Complete at least 10 to 20 reps.

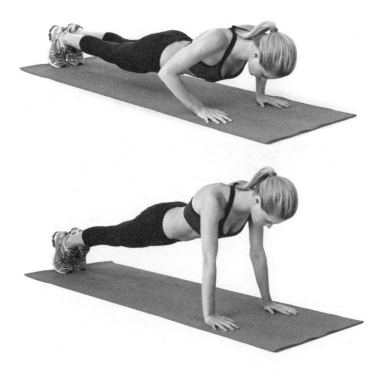

(continued)

THE PLANK

Remain in a push-up position, but instead of using your hands, rest your weight on your forearms. (Keep your elbows bent at 90-degree angles and pressed against the floor.) Keep your body straight, from your shoulders to your ankles. Suck in your abs, keeping your core tight throughout the exercise but making sure to breathe in and out. Hold the position for at least 20 seconds, gradually increasing the length of the exercise each time you do it. Without resting between them, do at least 2 reps in a period of 60 seconds.

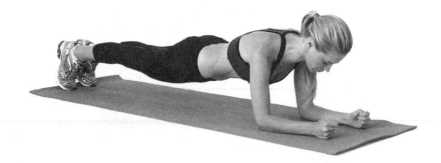

SQUATS

Stand with your feet about shoulder-width apart, then grab a dumbbell in each hand and hold them either at your sides or just above your shoulders. Contract your abs and hold them tight as you bend your knees and slowly squat down into a seated position; you should look as if you're sitting in an invisible chair, with your knees bent 90 degrees. Hold for 2 seconds, then contract your glutes and hamstrings as you lift up out of the invisible chair, extending your legs until you're standing. Do 8 to 12 reps, and shoot for 2 sets in a period of 1 minute. You'll maintain a similar position for the next exercise.

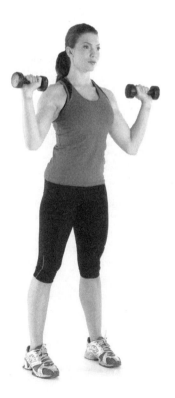
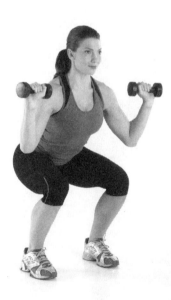

(continued)

THE BENT-OVER ROW

Stand with your feet shoulder-width apart and your knees slightly bent. Grab a dumbbell in each hand, then bend over until your back is almost parallel to the floor. With your arms in front of you and your palms facing in, slowly lower the dumbbells toward the floor and then pull them up on either side of your chest, making sure to squeeze the muscles in your back at the top of the movement. (This is a back-strengthening exercise.) Hold the weights at the top of the movement for a brief second as you contract your back muscles, then lower and repeat for 8 to 12 reps.

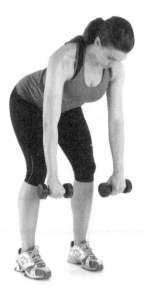 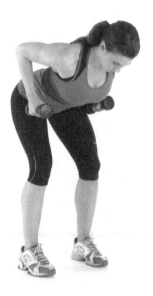

LYING TRICEPS EXTENSION

Lie face up on a padded floor or bench, extending your arms above your chest with a dumbbell in each hand. While keeping your upper arms steady and pointing straight up in the air, bend your elbows and lower the weights all the way down, stopping just as the weights are beside your ears. Raise the weights once again and, keeping your upper arms still, flex your triceps at the top of the movement. Try to do this without locking your elbows. Closing your eyes and concentrating on your triceps will help you target them and maintain proper form. Do 8 to 12 reps.

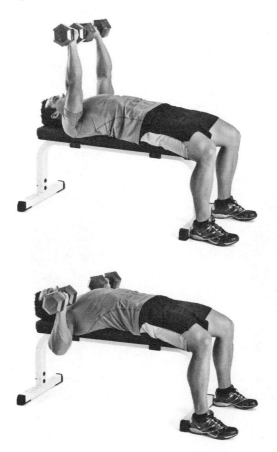

DUMBBELL CURLS

Grab your dumbbells with an underhand grip and hold them down in front of your thighs, palms facing forward. Keeping your upper arms steady, curl the dumbbells up toward your shoulders. At the top of the movement, squeeze your biceps—this is called a peak contraction, and it helps target and recruit your biceps for maximum burn. Feels good, doesn't it? Hold for a second after the brief contraction, then slowly lower the weights down to your thighs again and repeat for 8 to 12 reps.

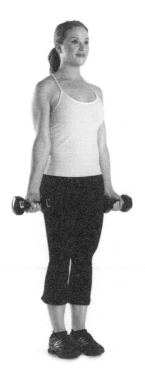
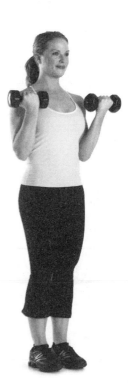

DUMBBELL SPLIT SQUATS

Stand with your feet shoulder-width apart. Hold your dumbbells at your sides and take a large step forward with your right leg. As you do this, press the front of your left foot into the ground and hold your balance. Lower your body straight down, keeping your back straight and your upper body upright, until your front knee is bent 90 degrees, your front thigh is parallel with the ground, and your back knee is just a few inches off the ground. Can you feel it in your glutes and your abs? Pause for a few seconds, then return to the starting position and repeat for 8 to 12 reps.

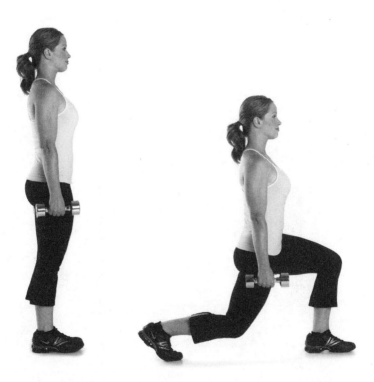

DUMBBELL SHOULDER PRESS

Stand or sit on a chair, holding your dumbbells at eye level with your arms out to the side, elbows bent at 90-degree angles, and your palms facing forward. Press the dumbbells straight up over your head, pausing at the top of the movement before slowly bringing the weights back down to the starting position. Lower the dumbbells to around ear level, making sure not to bring them down much further, which would put unnecessary stress on your shoulders. Do 8 to 12 reps.

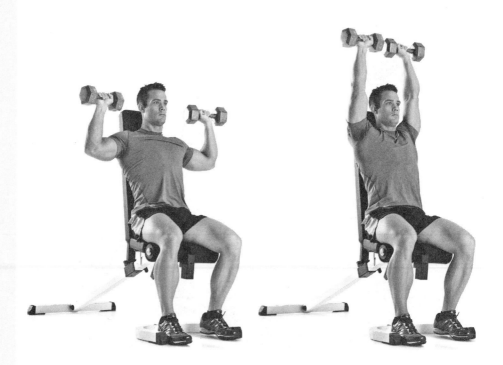

CRUNCHES

Now it's time to finish your circuit with some core work. Start by lying face up on the floor with your knees bent. Curl your shoulders toward your pelvis, keeping your hands crossed over your chest or beside your neck and making sure not to push against your head with your hands. Do 12 reps, then pop up and take a breather before you repeat the circuit.

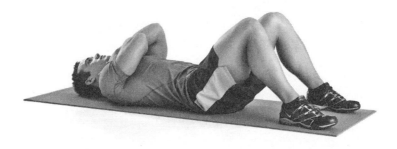

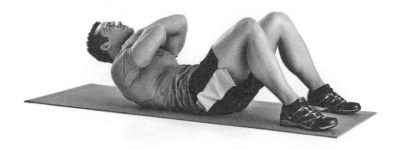

different exercises, one after another. For example, you might do a set of push-ups, followed by a set of bicep curls, followed quickly by a set of squats, and continuing on to other exercises that target every major muscle group. Once you're done with that "circuit," you take a rest and then repeat.

"It's nonstop movement for 45 minutes straight. It's like doing aerobics with weights. You're doing jumping jacks with weights. You're doing squats. It's constant movement of your body using weights. When I do 45 minutes of circuits, Lose It! says I burn 850 calories. It's pretty crazy."

Sean's high calorie-burn can be attributed to the fact that his workout includes circuit training in conjunction with interval training—a highly intense, effective combination.

"Doing circuits is known as high-intensity interval training (HIT). Your interval, instead of being a time period, is the muscle you're working out. I'm doing biceps for 30 seconds, then I'm going from biceps to legs, and after that I'm going to my shoulders for 30 seconds, and then I'm dropping down and doing my calves. So I'm never resting."

THE "NO-EXERCISE" EXERCISE PLAN

Okay, you know that when it comes to weight loss, exercise is essential. But what if now just isn't the right time for you to start an exercise plan? Do you have to wait months before you can reap the benefits of burned calories? Absolutely not.

With Lose It!, there is always a way to shed pounds if you have the motivation to do so. Even if you can't commit to hours of gym time every week, there are plenty of ways to get a little more physical activity into your day and burn some extra calories.

Stand Up for What You Believe In

When you think about how much time most of us spend sitting every day—excluding the 7 to 8 hours we typically sleep and the hour we might spend at the gym—it's pretty shocking. Between sitting at our desks during the day, sitting down for meals, sitting on our couches in the evening, and sitting in our cars at all hours, we easily spend 10 or more hours a day on our behinds. In fact, most of us spend more than *two-thirds* of our waking hours lounging around in one form or another.

Why is sitting such a big deal? Well, if you're trying to lose weight, sitting is one of the least-active things you can do with your body; it requires hardly any effort and expends almost no calories other than the energy required to maintain your vital signs. Put simply, the more time you spend on your seat, the larger it is likely to be.

The act of standing up requires far more energy than sitting and burns double the amount of calories. (This is your cue to stand up while you read, by the way.) When you stand, you support your own body weight, stabilize your back and core, and engage muscles from your legs to your core, all the way up to your shoulders.

A 155-pound person burns 36 calories sitting on the couch for 30 minutes and double that, about 73 calories, standing up for roughly the same amount of time. So start standing more often—give up your seat on the subway or bus, get up from your desk regularly at work, and the next time you're waiting for a train or plane, why not pass the time standing? You'll have plenty of time to sit soon enough.

Get NEAT to Lose

Standing is just one way to burn extra calories. When you think about it, there are lots of opportunities to burn calories every day. Scientists have termed this type of movement "non-exercise activity thermogenesis," or NEAT, and it refers to all of the energy you burn outside of traditional exercise.

An emerging line of research shows that NEAT accounts for why some people who don't exercise are obese and others who are seemingly just as sedentary are thin. The chart below illustrates just how much more energy you can expend through everyday NEAT activities.

When scientists at the Mayo Clinic conducted a study that compared the NEAT activities of nonexercisers—some lean, some obese—they found that the obese participants spent an extra 2½ hours sitting each day compared to their lean counterparts. The obese participants also expended

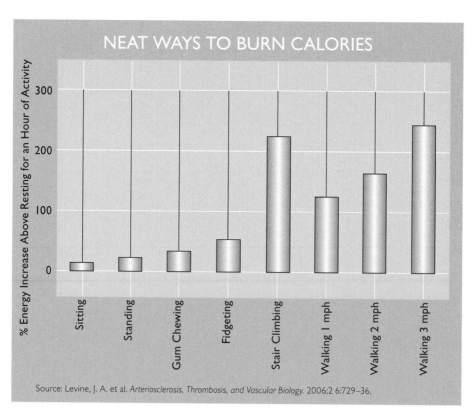

NEAT WAYS TO BURN CALORIES

% Energy Increase Above Resting for an Hour of Activity

Sitting, Standing, Gum Chewing, Fidgeting, Stair Climbing, Walking 1 mph, Walking 2 mph, Walking 3 mph

Source: Levine, J. A. et al. *Arteriosclerosis, Thrombosis, and Vascular Biology.* 2006;2 6:729–36.

about 350 fewer calories than the lean subjects during typical nonexercise activities such as working, commuting, and putzing around at home.

"Obesity was rare a century ago and the human genotype has not changed over that time," the Mayo Clinic researchers wrote. "Thus, the obesity epidemic may reflect the emergence of a chair-enticing environment to which those with an innate tendency to sit, did so, and became obese."

The thin participants in the study burned just 350 calories a day more than their obese counterparts. That number doesn't seem very significant, but over the course of several years, it can have a huge impact.

HOW AN EXTRA 350 CALORIES A DAY STACKS UP

In 10 days, that equals 3,500 calories, or 1 pound	In 30 days, that equals 3 pounds	In 6 months, that equals 18 pounds	In 1 year, that equals 36 pounds

Every Journey Begins with a Single Step

In 2009, scientists at a large hospital in Switzerland conducted a study published in the *European Journal of Internal Medicine.* The study examined the impact of daily activities on the body weight of a group of young doctors. None of the participants were overweight, and they all had similar jobs working in the same ward of a hospital. Yet the study found that some participants walked *four times* further than their peers on a typical day—2 miles, compared to 0.6 miles. And not surprisingly, the doctors who walked more during the day weighed less than their colleagues. The more active doctors weren't running laps around the pediatrics ward or hitting the gym at lunchtime; they just spent more time walking around.

Carol Redmon, a Lose It! user who works as a registered nurse at a hospital in South Carolina, understands this phenomenon well. When Carol started using Lose It!, she weighed 220 pounds and was eager to slim down and improve her overall health. In addition to tracking her calories and making better food choices, Carol also realized that she needed to burn more calories to reach her weight-loss goal.

"I work a 12-hour shift during which the activity level may fluctuate widely," she said. But Carol knew that little things add up, so she looked for simple ways to get more movement into her day, including parking at the edge of the lot so she had to walk further to the hospital entrance and walking up the stairs instead of taking the elevator. The result of all of those little changes? A big difference. To date, Carol has lost 40 pounds.

A 2008 study published in the *Journal of the American Medical Association* showed that people with high levels of nonexercise activity are just as likely to gain weight if they spend more time sitting down. This means that if a thin person reduces his or her activity level, they'll gain weight—and pretty rapidly, too. Researchers studied a group of men who normally walk a lot, taking about 10,000 steps a day (as measured by pedometers). The men were asked to reduce their daily steps from roughly 10,500 steps a day to about 1,340 steps and to keep all other variables (including diet) the same.

The results were astounding. After only 2 weeks, their metabolisms lowered, their levels of triglycerides (a type of fat found in the blood) shot up, and perhaps most disturbing of all, they developed 7 percent more fat around their abdomens. In only 2 weeks! Similar changes were seen in men who reduced their steps from 6,000 to 1,300 a day.

HOW YOUR STEPS ADD UP

The bottom line is that *any* kind of activity will help you lose weight. The trick is to make small changes that you can do every day.

If you're an office- or cubicle-dweller, you probably don't have the same freedom that someone like Carol does to add steps to her day. But just because you're deskbound doesn't mean you can't burn a few extra calories, too. In fact, when a study published in the journal *Diabetes Care* in 2008 compared a large group of office workers who sat for long periods of time, it found that those who took the most frequent short breaks—just to stand up and stretch or walk down the hall for a cup of water—had smaller waists and faster metabolisms than those who sat for the longest stretches of time without getting up.

If You Add	In 1 Day You Would Burn	In 1 Week You Would Burn	In 1 Month You Would Burn	In 6 Months You Would Burn	In 1 Year You Would Burn
1,000 extra steps	50 calories	700 calories, or 0.2 pounds	3,000 calories, or 0.9 pounds	18,000 calories, or 5.2 pounds	36,000 calories, or 10.3 pounds
2,000 extra steps	100 calories	1,400 calories, or 0.4 pounds	6,000 calories, or 1.7 pounds	36,000 calories, or 10.3 pounds	72,000 calories, or 20.6 pounds
4,000 extra steps	200 calories	2,800 calories, or 0.8 pounds	12,000 calories, or 3.4 pounds	72,000 calories, or 20.6 pounds	144,000 calories, or 41 pounds
6,000 extra steps	300 calories	4,200 calories, or 1.2 pounds	18,000 calories, or 5.1 pounds	108,000 calories, or 30.9 pounds	216,000 calories, or 61.8 pounds
8,000 extra steps	400 calories	5,600 calories, or 1.6 pounds	24,000 calories, or 6.9 pounds	144,000 calories, or 41.1 pounds	288,000 calories, or 82.2 pounds

While everyone's stride is different, on average it takes about 2,000 steps to travel 1 mile. At a casual pace, that burns roughly 100 calories.

You can bet that once the 2-week-long study was over and these men went back to their normal routines, their bodies began to return to normal, too. Our ancestors going back thousands and thousands and thousands of years spent most of their days on their feet—hunting, working in fields, or traveling from one place to the next over great distances. We're genetically programmed to be active, to be up on our feet and moving around most of the day. When you deprive your body of this basic activity, your metabolism slows and you store energy as fat.

In the same way that you've been making simple changes to your diet, look for everyday opportunities to make better calorie-burning choices. Opt for the stairs over the elevator, take a stroll to the mailbox instead of driving to the post office, walk your dog instead of letting him out, cook a nice dinner instead of ordering in, or do some housework instead of plopping down in front of the television. The Lose It! app can show you the calorie-burn estimates for dozens of these activities, from playing catch to doing home repairs, so you can easily track your estimated calorie-burn. These small changes are entirely doable, and they *will* make a difference. It all comes down to personal decisions: Do you get up and move it to lose it for a few minutes at a time, or do you sit back and miss your chance to burn off breakfast?

Exercise Machines: Can You Count On Calorie Counts?

Speaking of gadgets, those calorie counts displayed on the cardio machines at your gym may seem helpful, but if you're relying on them for an accurate gauge of your calories burned, you're making a mistake, as they're very rarely accurate.

The reason is simple: Cardio machines use a standard formula to calculate your rate of calorie burn. But they can't take into account your personal metabolism, not to mention a range of other variables, such as whether you're leaning on the handles or doing other things that minimize (or maximize) your effort. Plus, when a machine's been in the gym for a while, it suffers wear and tear that changes its levels of resistance and thus distorts the data.

As a result, most machines overestimate your calorie burn by 10 to 20 percent. That's important because many people rely on that number to tell them how much they've burned so they know how much they can consume.

If you're using one of the gadgets mentioned on pages 104 and 105, you won't have to worry about any of this because you'll have an accurate calorie gauge right on your arm. But if you don't have one of those devices, there are a few things you can do to get a more accurate picture of your calorie-burn. One popular strategy in the Lose It! community is to factor a 15 percent margin of error into the numbers on the screen. You can also offset the overestimation by entering a slightly lighter weight (5 to 10 pounds less than your actual weight) when the machine prompts you to input your information. And finally, you can use your perceived level of exertion to get a better idea of how many calories you're actually burning. So how do you figure out your perceived level of exertion?

If weight loss starts in the kitchen, then it follows a path through the gym. Starting an exercise program is never easy, but the reward of literally seeing results within a week is pretty gratifying. And as you burn calories, you'll be able to augment your calorie allowance, giving you flexibility and the opportunity to eat more of what you want.

SYNC UP TO TRIM UP

Losing weight is a journey of small steps—but you don't have to count every single one of them by yourself. With Lose It!, you have access to a calorie-burn database of virtually every exercise you can imagine, from badminton to yoga, walking to weightlifting, and even skydiving and of course, ahem, sex.

If you're serious about tracking your daily footsteps, it might be a good idea to invest in a pedometer. Any pedometer will keep track of your steps and help you burn some easy calories by calculating how far you walk in a typical day (which, in turn, will help you figure out when and how you can double, triple, or better yet quadruple your steps).

But just like Lose It! revolutionized calorie counting, a slew of new gadgets are modernizing get-fit gear. Here's a look at a few that are worth considering.

The Fitbit, $99

A pocket-sized pedometer—about the size of a money clip—that uses a 3D motion sensor to track your steps taken, distance traveled, and calories burned. And if you keep it on as you tuck into bed at night, it'll track your hours and quality of sleep, telling you how long it took you to fall asleep, how often you woke up, and how long you actually slept. Not bad, considering how important proper sleep is to weight loss. All of this information is uploaded to a Web site every time you walk by the device's wireless base station, and that information can then be plugged into the Lose It! app to give you an even more precise break-down of your data-driven diet.

The Bodybugg, $175 and up

The Bodybugg syncs up perfectly with Lose It! and is truly cool. About the size of a wristwatch, it wraps around your upper arm and uses a network of sensors to measure your motion, skin temperature, and heat flux, all of which together give you an accurate assessment of how many calories you're burning during any activity, from running to weightlifting to sitting on your couch reading a book. It may sound complicated, but if you want your precise exercise expenditure calculated down to the last calorie, this would be a good investment. (Before you plunk down your money, though, keep in mind that most members of the Lose It! community find that the Lose It! database gives them more exercise options and details than they could ever need.)

The Forerunner 110, by Garmin, $250

The Forerunner will calculate distance, calories burned, and, on top of that, heart rate. It's definitely not cheap, but over the long haul, those extra features that push up the price could end up bringing down your weight.

The Nike+ SportBand, $59

If the Forerunner 110 and Bodybugg are just too hard on your wallet, then you can find similar devices for less. The Nike+ SportBand wraps around your wrist and will measure your distance, pace, and calories burned. What's more, all you have to do to get that information on your computer is slide off the device's removable face and plug it right into your USB port. It's quick, easy, and affordable.

Pedometers, $4.99 and up

You can find any number of simple pedometers that won't break the bank, like the Ekho 3, which costs less than 20 bucks. At Target and other discount stores, you can even find pedometers for about 5 bucks. That said, sometimes it's worth it to spend the extra 5 or 10 dollars for something reliable and durable.

THE OFFICE OLYMPICS

Sneak in some stealth moves at the office to amp up your calorie-burn (and make work a little more interesting!).

Chair-Robics

Every time you stand in your cubicle for 5 minutes, you burn roughly 15 calories.

Stand up for 5 minutes every hour to stretch, talk on the phone, shuffle some papers around, or walk to the bathroom or water fountain for a quick break. Do that once every hour during an 8-hour workday, and you'll burn:

120 calories a day

600 calories a week

You'll lose **4.5 pounds** in 6 months, or about **9 pounds** in a year.

Climbing to the Top

According to research, every time you climb a single step, you burn about 0.1 calorie. When you walk down a step, you burn 0.05 calorie.

Try walking up three flights of steps, then walking back down and returning to your desk once every 2 hours at the office, and you'll burn:

20 calories a day

100 calories a week

You'll lose **0.8 pounds** in 6 months, or about **1.5 pounds** in a year.

Smoke Relays

What if you joined your friend every time he went out for a cigarette break—not to smoke, but to walk a couple of blocks?

The average person burns about 5 calories walking the length of one city block. Try walking around the block once while your friend is smoking. Do that three times a day and you'll burn:

60 calories a day

300 calories a week

You'll lose **2 pounds** in 6 months, or about **4 pounds** in a year.

Chapter Four

Do These Friends Make Me Look Fat?

Find Your Copilot on the Road to Weight Loss

Consider your social network for a moment.

Think about the people you see most often, the people you live with, the relationships that are most meaningful to you.

Now think about their body types.

Do they remind you at all—in shape and size, even in some small way—of yourself? According to the science of social networks, there's a good chance that they do.

We know this thanks in part to the good people of the small, close-knit New England town of Framingham, Massachusetts. That's where, in 2007, scientists from Harvard University and the University of California, San Diego, carried out a groundbreaking analysis of a large social network of more than 12,000 people.

The folks who took part in this landmark study were observed for more than three decades. They originally signed up to be part of a study on heart disease, but in order to keep tabs on their subjects, the researchers asked each of them to make a list of their friends and relatives. That way, there would be a record of people who could track them down if they ever left the area.

Keeping account of all these people allowed the scientists to gather a wealth of detailed information about the town's population, which they then used to construct a giant social web. Like hacking into a vivid and very active Facebook page, they could see how everyone was connected and how they changed over time—including how their weights evolved. What the scientists found was remarkable: People were most likely to put on weight when a close friend had also gained weight. In fact, when a friend became obese, it increased a subject's chances of becoming obese by up to 171 percent. And the closer the friend, the greater the risk. The same correlation could be made for weight loss, too, and distance made no difference. It didn't matter whether the friend lived a block away or moved across the country, the influence remained.

But this trend wasn't just the result of birds of a feather flocking together—thin people choosing thin friends, obese people taking comfort in other overweight confidants. The study revealed a psychological underpinning for this behavior: When a person packs on extra pounds, it makes being overweight seem more socially acceptable to their close friends. In other words, when your good friends are a little plump around the middle, you develop a subconscious acceptance of it. Suddenly, gaining a few pounds doesn't seem like such a crime—so bring on dessert!

But when your pals are losing weight, their skinny new physiques tend to make you feel a little more self-conscious about that extra weight you're lugging around town, and their healthy habits start to rub off on you. Your friend signed up for a yoga class? It might be fun to go with her. Your wife is cutting back on calories? Sounds like something you could get onboard with, too.

When you think about it, it's not that surprising. Humans are the most social creatures on Earth, and so many of our behaviors—both positive and negative—are easily influenced by the people around us. For good or bad, our behaviors and attitudes are just as contagious as a cold or flu virus.

In America, that influence has mostly been negative. As our neighbors have grown in size, so have we. But the results of the Framingham study offer proof that the opposite also holds true. All it takes is the determination to slim down—and asking for a little help from your friends.

FORGET ABOUT FACE TIME: FIGHT FAT ONLINE!

Achieving lifelong weight loss is certainly no easy feat. But there's an old proverb that sums up what many Lose It! users have discovered firsthand: No road is long with good company.

You can always choose to travel the road alone. But study after study has shown that tackling a challenge like weight loss with the support of friends or family dramatically increases your odds of success. As a 2-year study in the *Archives of Internal Medicine* showed in 2009, people who enroll in a diet and exercise program with at least one friend or relative lose nearly double the weight of those who try to lose weight on their own.

And nowadays you don't even need face time for the buddy system to work. A simple text, phone call, or e-mail message from a friend can be enough to keep you on track. In a 2009 study at the University of California, San Diego, overweight people who received a couple of supportive or encouraging text messages each day from their buddies lost almost *5 pounds more* than other dieters who didn't receive peer support.

You already have friends that you meet for dinner, drinks, or Monday Night Football—friends you celebrate with and friends you commiserate with when you're having a bad day. So why not enlist the help of your friends to lose weight? They'll thank you for it when they're 5 pounds thinner, too.

PEER PRESSURE WORKS

Peer support is one of the five pillars of the Lose It! philosophy. In this uberelectronic day and age, you're never more than an e-mail, tweet, or double-click away from your social network. Why not take advantage of technology to help you find instant motivators and support from a community of people who've "been there, done fat," and who can help you overcome the same hurdles they once faced? Here are a few ideas for finding support online.

Facebook

If you're like most people, you probably already spend hours every week clicking through photos, chatting with friends, and posting updates on Facebook. While you're there, why not lose some weight, too?

You can turn to your Friends list or visit the Lose It! Facebook page to find a wealth of knowledge, support, and information. You can even find people who are specifically looking for friends to support them as they lose weight (and friends for them to support, as well).

Loseit.com

The Lose It! forums (forums.loseit.com) are filled with people looking for friends, success stories, tips, and requests for help. If you're looking for someone with a set of goals similar to your own, that's where you'll find them.

In fact, Lose It! can automatically scan your e-mail address book and suggest friends who are already using the program. But Lose It! can also match you with people around the country who are similar to you (whether by age, weight, geography, weight-loss target, or interests).

SHARE YOUR JOURNEY

In order to benefit from your social network, you'll need to be open about your goals, progress, challenges, victories, and setbacks. By sharing your journey openly, your network will know when you're facing a struggle and need some help or when you've hit a milestone and could use a good cheer. Don't be bashful. We're all human, and we all need motivation, especially when it comes to weight loss. Here are a few ways you can communicate your weight-loss journey with others.

> You can use the Lose It! app to automatically update your Facebook wall or Twitter page when you exercise, set a new goal, weigh in, or hit a milestone. (That way, your support network is instantly notified about the details of your progress.)

> If you enjoy writing and aren't bashful about putting your life online, a blog can be a great way to share your weight-loss successes and struggles. You can set up a blog for free through a number of services. (Wordpress.com and blogger.com are two popular sites.) Just be aware that maintaining a blog requires a pretty substantial investment of time and energy.

> The Lose It! app can automatically send an e-mail summarizing your day or your week to anyone you'd like. Working with a trainer or nutritionist? Send him or her a summary of your workouts and food choices.

Have a spouse that's supporting your goal? Send her a daily summary to help control your craving for pizza night.

> Not using the Lose It! app? Then go to your Facebook page and update your status from time to time. Maybe you had a great workout, lost 2 pounds this week, or discovered a new low-calorie recipe that tastes amazing. Share your victories and tips and watch your motivation grow.

> Share your failures, too. This is harder, but just as crucial as sharing your successes. Support may be in the form of constructive feedback, a shoulder to cry on, or tips for getting past a plateau. You need your support group more than ever when you struggle.

> Follow your favorite blogs. Online weight-loss forums and blogs are popular places for people to share their successes and frustrations and to get support. Here are a few places where you'll find free and useful forums.

- Caloriecount.about.com

- Obesitydiscussion.com

- 3fatchicks.com

- Webmd.com

- Prevention.com/community/forums

THE SISTERHOOD OF THE SHRINKING PANTS

There's no question that peer support can help you pry off the pounds. In fact, Diana Bennett of Oklahoma is living proof of the effectiveness of peer support.

In 2008, Diana welcomed a bundle of joy into her life: her first grand-child. For Diana, 52, it was a blessing. She happily offered up her time for babysitting duty, spending hours in her rocking recliner holding her new granddaughter. But all of that sitting soon began to have an impact on her weight: She found herself exercising less and eating whatever was easiest to grab, which was often junk food. Diana had previously lost 50 pounds with Weight Watchers, but after 2 years of babysitting, half of that weight had crept back on.

"I gave up going to meetings to sit in the recliner with my grandchild," she says. "I just got tired of counting points and I stopped doing it. My grandchild is now 2 years old. In that 2 years, we both gained 25 pounds!"

Diana knew she needed an alternative, and after receiving an iPhone as a gift from her children, a friend told her about Lose It!

"Using Lose It! was a lot easier than Weight Watchers. Counting points is a part of the diet, but counting calories is a part of life. The simpler you can make it, the easier it is."

With Lose It!, Diana got back on track with her eating and lost 25 pounds. But one of her most crucial strategies was using the Lose It! Face-book page. She could benefit from social support any time of day—right from the comfort of her recliner and without taking her eyes off her granddaughter!

"When my granddaughter is napping, I can go on Facebook," she says. "I join the discussion board. I've met a lot of supportive people there. You make friends with people who don't necessarily want to talk about all of their problems in life, just their weight-loss struggles. These people can totally relate to your struggle. It takes an obsession with get-ting healthy to lose weight, just like it takes an obsession with eating to gain weight."

In fact, two of Diana's best friends, Michelle and Trish, are people she's never met face-to-face. The three women met on the Lose It! Facebook page and communicate almost daily, helping each other get past plateaus and setbacks and celebrating one another's accomplishments.

"Michelle's lost 46 pounds. Trish has lost a little more than 50. And I found out that Michelle lives just 45 miles away. We've never met in person, but when she reaches 50 pounds lost we're going to meet up."

Diana and her two online friends have become accountability partners. They have access to one another's food and exercise logs and can see when any of them is skating too close to the Red Zone or skipping out on exercise.

"When my friends see that I'm way over in the red, they send me an e-mail and ask what's going on. It helps you get focused again. It lets me know that they're concerned, and I don't want to be a bad example to them and they don't want to be a bad example to me. When you're having a bad day, you ask for their help, or if you're having an especially good day, then you can make their day better."

Having her friends hold her accountable—and vice versa—helped Diana so much that she became the Lose It! Facebook page's unofficial cheerleader. She visits the page daily and posts at least half a dozen times, usually congratulating someone on an accomplishment or offering advice when people are struggling. "It helps me to help others," she says. "If I preach it enough, it soaks in for me, too. If I can motivate others, then I can motivate myself."

In fact, if you put down this book and go online right now, there's a good chance you'll find Diana there, ready to welcome you to the community and offer a helping hand.

CREATING A NETWORK THAT WORKS

By now it should be clear: When it comes to losing weight (and most other things in life), having peer support makes a huge difference. Your peers can not only talk you through your impulse for a 3 a.m. ice cream binge, they can also inspire you to set new goals, such as running your first 5K or joining a weekly yoga class.

The key is to figure out what motivates you and then design a program around the people and the mechanisms that work for you specifically. *You* certainly aren't generic, and your social strategy for weight loss shouldn't be, either.

Throughout the rest of this chapter, you'll discover the many ways you can customize your social network and learn some of the strategies that have already worked for millions in the Lose It! community. It's up to you to decide which of these options are right for you.

Let's start with a few basic questions.

> Do you stick to a plan when you know that someone's keeping an eye on you, whether it's a trainer, a friend, a spouse, or a sibling? If so, you would probably benefit most from a **Keeping Tabs** support system.

> Are you motivated to succeed at weight loss (and anything else) because you want to do as well, if not better, than those around you? Then a **Friendly Competition** support system can help you reach your goals.

> Do you find that you're able to stay on track most of the time but need support on those rare occasions that you fall off the wagon? A **Safety Net** support system can help pick you back up.

> Do you enjoy spending time connecting with people but feel like you just don't have the time to fit socializing into your schedule? Then an **Online Connection** support system is probably your best bet.

Let's take a closer look at how each of these support systems can benefit you.

Keeping Tabs

Ask yourself: Would you stick to your plan if you knew that there was someone there to hold you accountable every time you dipped in for another spoonful of peanut butter? If you find yourself wandering into dangerous territory (like the cookie jar or ice cream tub) when no one is watching, it can be helpful to have someone who's looking over your shoulder, keeping tabs on your progress.

Lose It! user Donneen Kelley Parrott of Oklahoma credits her sister with helping her lose more than 40 pounds. Donneen asked her sister to follow her progress online, and she does, checking in regularly and sending Donneen text messages when she notices her sister slipping up. Donneen says that just knowing that someone is logging on and watching her progress day by day is motivation enough to stick with her game plan.

"Knowing that she's going to see whether or not I exercised, that's very motivating," says Donneen. It's like an accountability partner. If I haven't logged anything all day, she'll send me messages and ask why I haven't logged my food."

Even if you're not tracking your progress online, you can still ask a friend, colleague, or spouse to be your accountability partner. Ask them for what you need: If you want someone to send you texts once a day, express that. If you need someone to keep tabs on you more or less often, be sure to communicate how much "checking in" you're comfortable with. After all, there's a fine line between keeping tabs and policing—and the latter probably won't feel as positive and encouraging.

Friendly Competition

Competition isn't for everyone. But if you're the type of person who cranks up the speed on your treadmill to keep up with the jogger on the machine beside you, or who struts to the front of yoga class to get a better view in the mirror, let's face it: Competition is in your blood. So why not use that competitive spirit to your advantage?

Pick a workout buddy—someone who motivates you to lift a little more, run a little further, stay a little longer, work a little harder. Or, if you don't have a friend who goes to your gym, join a group class or sign up for a charity run or bike ride—sometimes even complete strangers can get your competitive juices flowing and motivate you to go the extra mile (literally).

You can also get competitive online. Make sure you and your friendly competitors have access to one another's food and exercise logs, and try to outdo—or at least keep up with—one another.

Lose It! user Brian Zamora of Seattle has lost 50 pounds, fueled, he says, by competition with his coworker. "There'd be times when I could see that my buddy went hiking for 4 hours and burned a lot of calories, and that would motivate me," Brian says. "If it was a Saturday where I wasn't doing anything and I saw him exercising, I'd think, 'I can't let him beat me!' So I'd go to the gym and do a bunch of cardio."

Some people are so competitive that they don't need another person to motivate them—they motivate themselves. If you're someone who's always looking to shave a few seconds off of your fastest mile or ratchet up

BE THE MOTIVATION YOU NEED!

Your social network is one way to stay motivated. But you can also draw motivation from within. In fact, a study by the Institute for Health Research and Policy in 2009 showed that regularly sending yourself encouraging tips and text messages could help you lose weight and maintain a slimmer waist. Messages like, "Only 8 pounds to go, keep it up!" will have a big impact.

Lose It! also allows you to set up alerts that remind you to keep logging. And you can send yourself e-mails or schedule exercise reminders on your electronic calendar. You can also choose to have weekly progress reports emailed to yourself and others in your social network, so you have even more reason to stay out of the Red Zone.

the leg press machine to the next notch, set small, achievable goals to keep your workouts challenging and your competitive juices flowing. And while you're feeling good about your accomplishments, why not brag a little? Be sure to update your Lose It! account with your latest achievements by clicking on the Motivators tab and linking your account directly to your Facebook or Twitter page. Diana says, "It's very motivating when you've been on the elliptical for 45 minutes and you post it on Facebook and other people click the 'Like' button."

As they say, a little friendly competition never hurt anyone. And—as Brian's story proves—it can certainly help you lose weight.

Safety Net

Let's say you're brimming with confidence. You've started logging, you're diligent, and you know you've got this weight-loss thing under control. It's so easy, it's so simple. You have no problem staying underbudget and you have no concerns about temptation getting the best of you. You're all set, right?

Not exactly. Doing the program alone is fine. But even if you have the discipline of a monk, you should still have a safety net in place, because you can never go wrong by planning for a rainy day. Plenty of Lose It! users have taken the lone-wolf approach but set up safety nets just in case they fall, and they've been thankful for it in the long run.

All you have to do is add a few friends to your list—personal acquaintances or weight-loss pals you've connected with online—and allow them access to your logs. You don't have to communicate with them on a daily or even weekly basis. But if you have an off week during which you stop logging, chances are they'll notice and will do what they can to get you back on track. Even the most determined, disciplined people sometimes stumble. When Sean Willson fell off the Lose It! wagon for a week, old friends in his network came out of the woodwork to give him the boost he needed.

"Four or five friends reached out to me and said, 'What happened?'," he said. "Their messages helped me. Even if I don't share everything with them all of the time, it's good to know that I have friends out there who are looking out for me."

If you're not using Lose It! online, you can set up safety nets for yourself in other ways. Ask a friend to check in with you weekly or monthly, whatever feels right to you. The important thing is to know that there's someone there to catch you—just in case.

Online Connection

Many people find that joining a weight-loss support group is highly effective. The only problem is, life can get in the way of any standing appointment, let alone your Thursday night weight-loss meeting. Long days at work, kids, visiting in-laws, bad weather . . . there are a million obstacles that can crop up on any given night. And soon you find that 1 or 2 weeks of playing hooky can make you reluctant to go back . . . and that starts to throw your progress in reverse.

If you want to reap the benefits of a weight-loss meeting without the hassle and inconvenience of having to be there in person, then start your own meetings online, at any time, on the Lose It! Facebook page or Loseit.com discussion boards. At any time of the day or night, there will always be someone else there, ready to chat.

Diana says she tried one weight-loss plan and liked the program but found it difficult to make the weekly meetings fit into her schedule.

"If you can't go to the Monday night meeting, you lose some of your motivation," Diana says. "With Lose It!, it's not, 'I have to be there on Monday night or I'm going to miss it.' I can get up at midnight, and instead of having a snack I can get online. Someone will be there and they can help me."

FANTASY WEIGHT-LOSS TEAM: DRAFT YOUR STARTING PLAYERS

Every successful team has a carefully crafted playbook and the right players to carry it out. Now that you've had a chance to consider various methods of social support, it's time to think about the players who'll get you to your goal. Lose It! users have identified three key teammates that help them stay on track.

1. The Healthy Cooking (and Eating) Partner. The kitchen is a major battlefield in the war on fat. For many in the Lose It! community, it's also where weight loss begins. People who lose 50 pounds or more often do it with a partner who changes his or her diet, too, and who adopts a newer, healthier approach to cooking and dining out.

If you rely on your husband, wife, parent, or someone else to do most of the cooking and grocery shopping in your home, then that person has a big influence on your progress. Ask him or her for the support you need. Explain which foods you're cutting back on or eliminating from your diet, and suggest lower-calorie alternatives and recipes. When eating out, recommend restaurants that have a wider array of low-calorie options.

Brian Newby of Florida lost over 100 pounds with Lose It!, but his most important turning point came when his wife, Melissa, got on board with the program.

"My wife took it as a challenge to cut calories. She's always been a great cook, but she started to make meals for the whole family that were both healthy and low-calorie. She would cook meals and divide them into individual portions. This led to a lot of leftovers, which turned into lunches for us throughout the workweek. Slowly, we both learned what we could eat reasonable portions of and what would weaken our resolve. We frequented restaurants that published their nutritional data. If we couldn't figure out what we were eating, we wouldn't eat it."

The reality is, you might have to change your habits for a while. If you have friends that meet for taco or steak night and you can't stand to be in a restaurant with so many unhealthy options, then create a new option. You could suggest trying a different restaurant, invite your buddies over for dinner and cook something a bit healthier, or simply skip your standing night out and meet up with friends who want to do something active.

2. The Gym Buddy. Even Olympic athletes—motivated, disciplined overachievers—often train as part of a team. No matter how much devotion you have to your new workout plan, there will be times when it would help to have a few teammates. As a study conducted by the Stanford Prevention Research Center showed, support that's specific to exercise is a far better predictor of exercise adherence than general social support.

The right gym buddy can motivate you to go to the gym and kill it while you're there. You might even plan a reward for after your workout, like grabbing a bite together at your favorite lunch spot.

Who would make the best gym buddy? Here are some guidelines to consider before you choose.

> **Find a workout partner with similar goals.** If your target weight is 80 pounds away, then a friend with only 20 pounds to go probably won't be the kind of wingman you need.

> **Look for a person who likes a good challenge.** This is a person who's not afraid to get her heart rate up, who's always game to try out a new activity, and who will push you to pick up the pace when your legs feel like they're made of lead.

> **Recruit someone who enjoys the same activities.** Pick a buddy with similar exercise interests, then sign up to take a class together—spinning, step aerobics, kickboxing, Zumba—something you can both get excited about. Besides the fun of doing it together, you'll have a standing commitment neither one of you will want to break, and if one of you has a tough time with the workout, the other will be right there to help.

3. The Inspirational Buddy. Lasting weight loss is a long journey, and there will be times along the road when you stall. You'll be exercising, eating right, and watching your portion sizes, and you still might find yourself questioning your progress. You'll hit plateaus. You'll lose some steam. You'll find that if you're trying to lose 60 pounds, the first 30 will come off twice as easily as the last 30. (And by the way, that's totally normal.)

Whether it's online or in person, know which member of your team you can look to for inspiration. Maybe it's someone who's already lost a significant amount of weight, a friend who has dealt with life's challenges with grit and determination, or an uberfit buddy who has become a role model for you. This is the person who, when you can't go on any longer—run another mile, swim another lap, lift another rep, or even go to the gym at all—helps you get your second wind.

((()))

Lose It! encourages you to inject a little fun into weight loss. So why not earn a badge for your accomplishments? When you or one of your friends hits a weight-loss milestone, like losing 10, 20, or 50 pounds, you'll join the milestone club and earn a badge (see some examples on the opposite page).

If you run 20 miles in a week, set a new record with weekly visits to your gym, or accomplish some other achievement, it won't go unnoticed in the Lose It! community. Have a little tongue-in-cheek fun with your network to reinforce their good behaviors. You might be surprised at some of the fun rewards that can come your way. Nominate your friends for badges when they're doing well. Losing weight really is a big deal, and every milestone is worth celebrating. So go on and have a little fun!

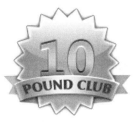
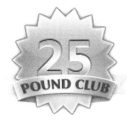
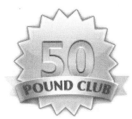
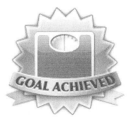
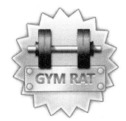
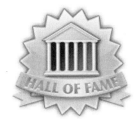

LOSE IT! FOR THE LITTLE ONES

As the Framingham study (page 108) illustrated so vividly, a change in one person's habits can push the collective body weight of an entire community in the wrong direction.

If you have children, then every decision you make at the grocery store, in a restaurant, or in your own kitchen has a direct effect on their waistlines. Their health is at the mercy of your food decisions—and today, that is more important than ever.

That's because the obesity crisis has affected the youth of our country even more than it has adults. In the past 30 years, the number of obese children has more than tripled, causing an entire segment of the adolescent population to have conditions that a few decades ago were unheard of in children: high blood pressure, high cholesterol, even heart disease. One study of 5- to 17-year-old children found that 70 percent of obese youth had at least one risk factor for cardiovascular disease!

Make no mistake, childhood obesity and adult obesity have the same root cause: overeating. That's not to suggest that you put your kids on a diet. But oftentimes when Lose It! users become more conscious of their own calories and food choices, their entire family reaps the benefits. Whatever you're eating at home, your kids are most likely eating, too—and they mimic your behaviors and attitudes, as well. In fact, parents' and children's diets are so intertwined that a 2009 study in the *International Journal of Obesity* showed that obese moms are 10 times more likely to have obese daughters, and obese dads are 6 times more likely to have obese sons.

The example you set for your kids can have more of an impact than you realize. Edward Clark of Indiana, who lost more than 60 pounds with Lose It!, raised his son on typical American kids' fare, never denying him the chicken fingers, mac 'n' cheese, and other empty calories that all children love. But one day he realized his son was following in his food-related footsteps.

"One day we were out at a restaurant, and instead of getting chicken fingers, he ordered the grilled chicken—and it was a choice that he made! That's when it kind of hit me and my wife that hey, the good choices we make really are having a positive impact on our kid."

In Edward's case, the positive changes trickled down to his son. But sometimes it takes a wake-up call in order to make a change, which is exactly what happened to Jennifer Mueller Krause of Washington.

Jennifer lost more than 35 pounds with Lose It! by controlling her portion sizes, exercising, and replacing soda and junk food with more satisfying snacks like Greek yogurt and fruit. But for a while, Jennifer didn't give much thought to her 3-year-old daughter's eating habits, allowing her to constantly munch on high-fructose corn syrup–laden "kid snacks." Then one day she took her daughter to the dentist. After her daughter's examination, the dentist informed her that her 3-year-old's teeth were so badly destroyed from decay that she needed to have two molars removed. Jennifer was horrified. She realized something that many Lose It! parents eventually discover: The changes you make to your own diet can easily be made to your children's diets, as well. Jennifer had already cut junk food out of her own diet and replaced it with healthy alternatives. Since those options were already in the house, there was no reason she couldn't encourage the whole family to eat healthier foods.

"Now we've all switched over to organic milk and organic peanut butter, and we've gotten rid of as much high-fructose corn syrup as we can. I realized that I was taking such good care of myself and not taking care of my daughter. But now her habits have changed. She asks for a banana for breakfast instead of Fruit Roll-Ups. And my husband is getting on the bandwagon, too!"

One family member's habits can inspire an entire household. Be a healthy example for your loved ones, then get your family in on it as well, for their own good. Don't assume that your kids won't eat a piece of fruit simply because they're used to Froot Loops and sugary snacks. So many Lose It! parents have phased healthy foods and low-calorie alternatives into their household diet. You don't have to eliminate every cookie and chip, but you can show your kids how to strike a healthy balance—just as you've done with your own diet. After all, improving your family's health is one more reason to stick with your own program.

Chapter Five

What's Your Type?

Identify the Habits That Are Holding You Back

It's true that no two people are alike. We are all individuals, unique as snowflakes (and as "special" as our parents always told us we were). But when it comes to food, we exhibit some surprisingly common behaviors.

So what's your type? Your *eating* type, that is.

When the kids are in bed, the last dish has been washed, and the day's events are replaying in your mind as you sit back and watch the evening news, do you instinctively reach for a pint of Häagen-Dazs, a glass of wine, or a good book and a cup of tea? When the long workweek is over and the weekend is *finally* here, do you stick to your budget as diligently as you did Monday through Friday, or do you take a minivacation and indulge your way straight into the Red Zone? Do you tell yourself you're just going out for coffee but end up coming back—time after time, despite your best efforts—with a sugary snack that wrecks your calorie budget? (That darn scone again!)

These habits are probably a large part of the reason why you gained weight in the first place. And even now, as you're fighting hard to make better decisions and lose the pounds, those habits can sneak back into your life and sabotage your efforts.

But you're not doomed to repeat the mistakes of the past—you can change the habits that challenge your best weight-loss intentions and even create new habits that will set you up for success. Lose It! has helped millions of people discover their belt-busting behaviors *and* take control of them. The reality is, recognizing your own personal, problematic eating patterns is a crucial part of not just losing weight, but also keeping it off for good. You have to know your weaknesses and vulnerabilities if you're going to be able to save yourself from giving in to them. After all, if you're working hard to make better choices and stay under your calorie budget 85 percent of the time, but your weight loss is undermined by the way you behave the other 15 percent of the time—well, that's enough to sap just about anyone's motivation.

Luckily, Lose It! can show you how to identify the patterns that push you into the Red Zone. If you stop and think about it, using Lose It! is essentially like conducting a giant case study of a single person's dietary choices, patterns, behaviors, and trouble spots. And that person, of course, is *you*.

After only a week of faithfully logging your food, you'll already have accrued a mound of data that, if you take the time to analyze it, will reveal everything you need to know about the way you eat, exercise, and make decisions. Review this information to find common themes—patterns of behavior that are consistent over time. Once you've connected the dots and identified the patterns that are causing you to plateau or gain weight, you can implement a personalized solution.

CHARLES IN CHARGE

One person who is intimately familiar with the powerful insight you can gain from analyzing your eating patterns is a man who's been using Lose It! literally since day one. His name is Charles Teague, and in addition to being one of the authors of this book, he's also the founder and creator of Lose It!

Charles is just another guy trying to control his weight without relying on tricks or gimmicks. As a busy, hardworking family man whose weight has fluctuated throughout his adult life (from a low of 185 pounds on his wedding day to a high of 215, back in the days when he subsisted on a software programmer's diet of pizza and Mountain Dew), his goal is simply to get back to his fighting weight.

But more than a few temptations stand in his way, and somewhere near the top of that list are two of his favorite things on Earth: freshly brewed coffee and glazed donuts. As luck would have it, Charles lives only two blocks away from a coffee shop. But unfortunately for Charles, that coffee shop just happens to be Dunkin' Donuts.

"It's like the universe has conspired against me," says Charles. "When I stop and get a cup of coffee on the way to work, the donuts are right there! And if I'm running late that day, I think, 'Oh, I'll just grab a donut for breakfast. It's easy.'"

Donuts, of course, are not exactly a low-calorie food. One Dunkin' Donuts Glazed Cake Stick and a large cup of coffee can easily set Charles back 400 calories before he even makes it to the office. Charles created Lose It! as a way to tackle weight loss from an engineer's standpoint: Track everything you eat, and make sure what goes in is less than what goes out.

But it didn't take a scientist to see that, in Charles's weekly food logs, his morning Dunkin' Donuts run was swallowing up a giant chunk of his daily calorie budget and driving him further and further from his goal. It was clear something had to be done. Skipping Dunkin' Donuts altogether was out of the question—Charles loves their coffee, and it's the closest place to his house.

"My first strategy was just to choose a lower-calorie item. I traded down from a Glazed Cake Stick to a Glazed Donut," he says.

That took him from 340 calories per trip down to about 220 calories—a savings of 120 calories a day. But pretty soon, he found that this strategy wasn't working. One donut just wouldn't cut it.

"The problem became that I wasn't that satisfied after a Glazed Donut, so I'd want to get a couple of them, and then I'm up to 450 calories for breakfast and I'm still hungry by midmorning. It's not a good breakfast, and I know that for the rest of the day I'm going to have a problem because I've already used a lot of calories that don't even fill me up.

"I also found that eating the donuts would put me at a psychological disadvantage because then I would tell myself, 'I already blew it, so who cares what I eat for lunch? Since this day is a wash anyway, I might as well get a cheeseburger.'"

Charles's food log clearly reflected that those daily trips to Dunkin' Donuts were sabotaging his progress. He realized that if he just gave up his donut run, he could eat pretty well throughout the rest of the day and still have plenty of calories left for a healthy dinner with his wife. So Charles reassessed his budget, thinking of another way to fix it as an engineer would. The easiest calories to eliminate—the lowest hanging foods in his daily budget—were the ones from Dunkin' Donuts. They simply had to go.

"I realized that before I walked in the door at Dunkin' Donuts to get my coffee, I just had to tell myself that I wasn't going to get a donut. It's not like I'm surrounded by donuts all day. If I could just survive those 2 minutes, I'd be fine."

For someone else, sticking with one Glazed Donut might have worked. But for Charles, it didn't. Going cold turkey 5 days a week was the only solution. And so far, it's working. Once in a while he'll treat himself to a family donut outing on the weekend, but Monday through Friday is a no-donut zone.

Charles also learned something important about his eating "type" through this exercise in donut rehab: He craves sweets in the morning, and if he doesn't satisfy his sweet tooth to some degree, he's just not going to feel satisfied, period. His solution?

"I eat a bowl of kids' cereal (the really sweet stuff) in the morning before I leave to get my coffee," he says.

It may not be the breakfast of champions, but caloriewise, it's certainly a better choice than donuts. With ½ cup of skim milk, it's also more filling than a donut—and it satisfies Charles's morning sweet tooth.

Charles's Calorie Compromise

Having This for Breakfast	Instead of Having This	Saves Him	Over 5 Days, That Equals	Over 6 Weeks, That Equals
¾ cup of Frosted Flakes with ½ cup of skim milk (200 calories)	2 Glazed Donuts from Dunkin' Donuts (440 calories)	240 calories a day	1,200 calories	More than 2 pounds of weight gain avoided!

DETERMINING YOUR TYPE

Charles's story is a good example of why one-size-fits-all diets don't work. On almost any other diet, he would have been forced to give up his sweet breakfast craving entirely—but Charles just can't stomach the thought of a sugar-free breakfast. So he created a personalized strategy for his biggest dietary pitfall.

After analyzing the data of hundreds of thousands of Lose It! users, it's clear that many people share similar food struggles and behavior patterns. Those patterns can be grouped into five basic eating types. Chances are, you will identify with one or more of these behavior patterns. Once you identify your type (or types), you'll be able to develop strategies and solutions tailored specifically to your needs, whether that means steering clear of glazed donuts for breakfast or making better choices at happy hour.

Type #1: The Weekender

Are you someone who lives "by the book" all week, only to throw that book out the window on Friday night? Do you diligently log every last morsel of food that crosses your lips from Monday morning through Friday afternoon but then, as soon as you punch out at the office and make it to happy hour, forget that the free chips contain costly calories?

Or maybe you travel a lot for work or pleasure, and as soon as your surroundings change, so do your eating and food-logging habits. (Do calories still count when they're consumed in a different area code? Yes, they do.)

In 2010, Lose It! conducted a detailed study of user habits, selecting a random sample of 10,000 users and analyzing their eating patterns across a typical week.

The pattern that emerged was crystal clear: Most people start off the week strong but lose steam by Friday, culminating their week in a food fest that undermines their diligent efforts during the workweek.

Logging Your Food, Day by Day

The graph below illustrates (in blue) the percentage of Lose It! users who log their foods on each day of the week.

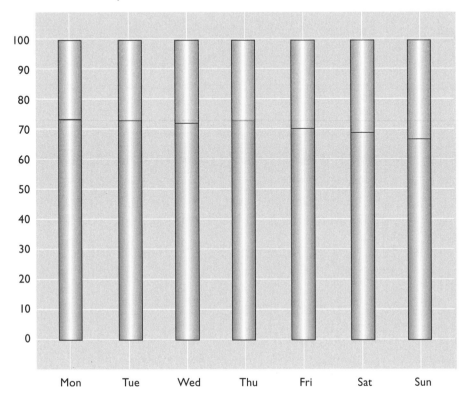

As you can see from the graph above, more than 70 percent of Lose It! users consistently log their foods between Monday and Thursday. But when the weekend rolls around, their logging becomes more sporadic. And by Sunday, they've hit rock bottom. Then, first thing Monday morning, all those guilt-ridden people who stopped tracking over the weekend are back at the kitchen table logging their breakfasts . . . and the cycle begins again.

But it's more than a matter of simply logging your food. Even those who *do* log on Saturday and Sunday tend to come down with a major case of weekenditis. Friday, Saturday, and Sunday are the days that people most frequently go overbudget and end up in the Red Zone. Friday and Saturday are particularly problematic, with more than 20 percent of users going overbudget on these two days (see the graph on page 136 for details).

No one wants to deprive you of a little R & R on the weekends, but consider for a moment how much fun those weekends will be when you're back in shape. Wouldn't you rather show up at the beach and feel confident enough to take off your shirt? Or have the stamina to go on a long hike, ski all afternoon, or just simply look smokin' hot in a cocktail dress or well-cut suit at a wedding? By all means, you should enjoy your weekends, but you can't expect to lose weight if you go *completely* off the reservation every single Friday at 5 p.m. To help keep you on track, here are a few damage-control strategies that don't require you to give up your weekend fun.

Splurge, baby, splurge. It's hard to resist going nuts on Saturday when you've been buttoned up for 5 days straight. But if you manage to inject a little food-related fun into the weekdays, you'll be less likely to "reward" your good weekday deeds with major damage on the weekends. So consider working one splurge night into your week. On your splurge night, you can have whatever you want for dinner—whether that's a burger, lasagna, pepperoni pizza, or French fries and a milkshake. Sure, it'll probably push you over your budget for the day, but it's better to have a single splurge than a three-day bender. Plus it'll give you something to look forward to each week. Sean Willson, a computer programmer in Illinois, lost more than 100 pounds with Lose It!, and a Friday night splurge is one way he keeps himself in line.

"I used to do free *days,* but that didn't work out. You end up going too far. So now I do a free *meal.* Every Friday I eat whatever I want for dinner. So if I've been craving pizza all week, I have pizza. If I'm craving steak, I'll

Out on the Town and Overbudget

The graph below illustrates (in blue) the percentage of Lose It! users who stay within their calorie budgets for each day of the week.

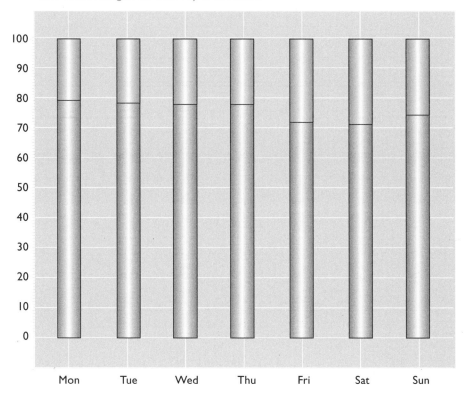

have a really nice steak and a baked potato. I always have a dessert, too. I feel like I've earned it. Food is no longer this thing that's destroying me. I reward myself with one great meal and I'm satisfied."

Make your everyday meals more exciting. If one splurge night a week just won't cut it, then spread some splurging across the week. Don't deny yourself good food—but indulge in moderation. Eat right up to the red line every day. If you're not looking forward to having a salad for lunch, go for a moderate portion of something you really want—maybe half of a high-calorie sandwich from your favorite shop. Or go ahead and have the salad for lunch, but add 150 calories' worth of feta cheese or lean protein to make it that much more satisfying. Make your most boring meals a little more exciting without going overboard. If the foods you eat during the week are more satisfying, you'll be less likely to fly off the calorie handle when the weekend rolls around.

Create the same experience with fewer calories. You can still have drinks and chips at happy hour, cake and ice cream at your kid's birthday party, and a hearty Saturday morning breakfast. But you can easily trim some calories from your favorite occasions by making wiser choices. As discussed in Chapter 2, trimming calories is really about making smart swaps; sometimes you just have to get a little creative. Instead of drinking three glasses of white wine on Friday night, sub in a couple of vodka sodas or another lower-calorie alternative. Instead of throwing the usual pancakes and sausages onto your plate on Saturday morning, pick some equally satisfying but lighter breakfast treats. You won't feel deprived, and it'll pay off in the long run. (See "Party Hard, Stay Slim" on page 138 for a few ideas to get you started.)

Travel smart. When you're on the road, you're out of your comfort zone and don't always have access to your go-to foods. Just try to make the best choices you can from what's available to you, and always keep an eye on portion sizes and look for ways to skim calories from a heavy meal. You might even pack some of your favorite low-cal snacks to take with you so that you'll have a go-to treat when you're feeling peckish. And don't stop logging just because you're away from home. If you have trouble staying within your calorie budget, squeeze in some exercise while you're away. Go for a quick workout in the hotel gym or do 20 minutes of sit-ups, push-ups, or other exercises in your room. If you're staying at a resort, take a break from lying in the sun to swim a few laps in the pool. Or go on a 45-minute walk into town, keeping a decent enough pace to

PARTY HARD, STAY SLIM

If You Like This	Then Try This	You'll Save	After 10 Weekends, That Equals
White wine, 4 ounces (90 calories); 4 glasses per weekend	Vodka soda (65 calories)	25 calories	Almost 0.3 pound
Rum and Coke, 2 ounces rum, 4 ounces cola (176 calories); 4 drinks per weekend	Rum and Diet Coke (128 calories)	48 calories	More than 0.5 pound
Ruffles Original potato chips, 24 chips (320 calories)	Baked! Lay's Original potato chips, 30 chips (240 calories)	80 calories	About 0.3 pound
Duncan Hines Moist Deluxe Classic Yellow Cake Mix, 1 serving (270 calories)	Pillsbury Moist Supreme Classic Yellow Cake Mix, 1 serving (230 calories)	40 calories	0.3 pound (assuming 2 slices per weekend)
Aunt Jemima Original pancakes, four 4-inch cakes, with 2 Tbsp maple syrup and 2 Jimmy Dean Breakfast Sausage Patties (610 calories)	Hungry Jack Buttermilk Complete pancakes, three 4-inch cakes, with 1 Tbsp maple syrup and 2 Banquet Brown 'N Serve Original Sausage Links (330 calories)	280 calories	Almost 1 pound
BurgerKing Whopper Value Meal (includes medium fries and medium Coca Cola) (1,160 calories)	BurgerKing Whopper Jr., side salad with fat free ranch dressing, water (450 calories)	710 calories	More than 2 pounds
Haägen-Dazs Chocolate Peanut Butter ice cream (360 calories)	Breyers All Natural Vanilla and Chocolate ice cream (130 calories)	230 calories	About 0.7 pound

burn 100 calories. Every little bit helps. And don't forget to log your exercise, too, so you can see the rewards.

Type #2: The Calorie Drinker

How many calories a day do you guzzle? One of the biggest food mistakes people make is thinking that if it's something you can sip, the calories won't stick. Unfortunately, liquid calories are stealth fatteners—they go down quickly, making it easy to drink more than your share of extra pounds. In fact, studies show that the average American gets almost 25 percent of his or her daily calories from beverages alone! That's nearly double the amount of calories we were imbibing daily 40 years ago.

Do you run out for coffee and come back clutching a large milkshake with a shot of caffeine? Starbucks may call it a Peppermint White Chocolate Mocha, but it's really a calorie bomb in coffee clothing: 470 calories, in fact. Or maybe soda is your downfall. According to the California Center for Public Health Advocacy, the average American consumes 50 gallons of soda a year—the equivalent of one and a half cans of soda each day. And let's not forget about all of those bottled teas and sugary sports drinks, and perhaps one of the most deceptively named beverages of all time—Vitaminwater. (It should really be called Sugarwater, as one bottle contains roughly 32 grams of the white stuff.)

But Vitaminwater is certainly not alone in the deceptively fattening drinks category. If you frequent Jamba Juice thinking you're getting a healthy snack, you may want to take a closer look at the nutrition labels. Smoothies can be a healthy option, but make the wrong choice and you're drinking a few extra pounds. According to Jamba Juice, when you order a Mango-a-go-go smoothie, "You'll feel great knowing you're getting antioxidants like vitamin C and beta-carotene (vitamin A)." But we bet you won't feel so great knowing that a large one of these packs 121 grams of sugars—that's 29 teaspoons' worth and 570 calories! Jamba Juice says its Strawberry Surf Rider will put some "pep in your step and a smile on your face." Order a large one with a whey protein boost just three times a week and it'll also slap 28 pounds onto your hips over the course of a year. Maybe you love to gulp down a large Peanut Butter Moo'd smoothie (770 calories) three times a week, but you're probably less excited about hitting the gym to work off the half pound of weekly weight gain it'll cost you.

Last but not least, there's the ultimate liquid calorie pitfall: alcohol. It's easy to forget that the five or six beers you sipped while watching the game on Sunday or the half bottle of wine you downed at your last book club meeting easily amounted to half of your calorie budget for the entire day!

Whether your weakness is coffee, soda, or cocktails, there's always a way to alter your drink of choice so it doesn't destroy your calorie budget and sabotage your progress.

Take it from Kent Metschan of Texas, who's lost about 50 pounds using Lose It!, in part by cutting calories from his favorite drinks: soda and Grande Caffè Mochas at Starbucks. Kent loves Coke, but now when he goes to his local sandwich joint in Austin, he gets a large fountain soda with a personal twist: He fills three-quarters of the cup with Diet Coke and then adds a splash of regular Coke on top.

"You can't even tell the difference!" he says.

In the past, Kent would chug a whopping 360 calories every time he ordered one of his Grande Caffè Mochas at Starbucks. Now he gets skim milk instead of whole milk, and he skips the whipped cream. Those two little changes save him almost 200 calories a cup! As the chart below illustrates, eliminating 140 calories each time you grab a cup of joe can have a huge impact over the long haul.

Kent's Favorite Drink Swaps, or "Large Coffee, Hold the Calories"

Kent Used to Order	Now He Orders	That Saves Him	After 8 Weeks, That Equals
A large Coca-Cola soft drink at Jimmy John's (400 calories)	Three-quarters Diet Coke, one-quarter Regular Coke (100 calories)	300 calories a drink	16,800 calories (1 drink per day), or about 5 pounds
A Grande Caffè Mocha at Starbucks (360 calories)	The same drink, but with skim milk instead of whole milk and no whipped cream (220 calories)	140 calories a drink	7,840 calories (1 drink per day), which is more than 2 pounds

Jennifer Zervos of Oklahoma used to indulge in sugary drinks, as well. But now she's lost more than 14 pounds by making some clever drink substitutions.

"I used to drink two bottles of soda every day, sometimes more. Now I drink water and an occasional Diet Dr Pepper, because it tastes like regular," she says.

Anthony Robertson is also a reformed Calorie Drinker, but his drink of choice was beer. He lives in Pennsylvania and loves the local stuff, Yuengling Traditional Lager. But a single bottle will set him back about 140 calories, so he found two awesome alternatives: Yuengling Light Lager, which has only 99 calories, and Michelob Ultra, which has a mere 73 calories per bottle. By making these changes and others, Anthony has lost more than 55 pounds.

"In the past I was drinking regular Yuengling, and that's just loaded with calories. I can have two Michelob Ultras for that one lager."

Anthony's Belly-Shrinking Beer Swaps

Anthony Used to Drink	Now He Drinks	That Saves Him	If He Drinks 2 Beers a Week for 10 Weeks, That Equals
Yuengling Traditional Lager (140 calories)	Yuengling Light Lager (99 calories)	41 calories per bottle	820 calories, or 0.25 pound
	Michelob Ultra (73 calories)	67 calories per bottle	1,340 calories, or more than 0.3 pound

Type #3: The Low-Hanging Food Grabber

Food, glorious food—everywhere you turn! Like all animals, our instinct is to grab any source of calories that comes our way—and if you're like Charles, sometimes those calories come in the form of donuts. These days we're confronted with calories everywhere we go, from bagels in the conference room to king-size chocolate bars in the checkout aisle (at the electronics store, no less).

In an environment with such an abundance of cheap, easy calories, temptation lurks at every corner. Sure, you start off each morning with the right attitude, but soon you're faced with tempting options that chip away at your willpower. After all, how can you refuse that slice of cake at your boss's birthday party when it's literally handed to you?

If these scenarios sound familiar, you need a strategy to overcome the allure of low-hanging foods. You can't expect to lose weight if you give in to these goodies every time, or even most of the time. At some point you have to make a compromise: I'll eat the small brownie on the catering tray, but not the giant cookie. Or I'll skip the free cake at the office now and when I get home, I'll have a bowl of the Cherry Garcia frozen yogurt that's in my freezer.

When you enter a dicey situation with a plan of action already in place, you'll have a better chance of resisting temptation (most of the time, at least), and you won't derail your weight loss. Fortunately, plenty of Lose It! users have found creative ways to moderate their "low-hanging" behaviors and reach their goals. If this is your eating type, here are a few helpful strategies.

Vigilance is a virtue! It's always important to track your meals, but in this case, it's extra important that you track every little bite. Up until now, you probably haven't been "counting" all those free samples at Starbucks, but they can easily cost you 100 calories or more. Just seeing how all of those extra bites add up is motivation enough to make you say no to the free muffin sample.

Plan for the unexpected. It's easier to indulge in the unexpected cookies, bagels, chips, and cake that life throws your way when you've already set aside some room for them. In other words, plan for the unexpected. If you know you're going to a party with a decadent spread, eat before you go so you're not standing by a pile of cookies while your stomach growls in protest. Then, use a small plate to taste a bit of the things you want the most. If you have your eye on the office party cake, find a colleague who's also trying to lose weight and split a slice between you.

Jeff Loats of Colorado has lost 20 pounds using Lose It! But Jeff is a low-hanging food grabber, and to reach his target, he had to cope with constant temptations.

"Home is probably the toughest place for me, especially if I'm home all day. I tend to wander into the kitchen and grab things if they're visible or easily available. I'm especially a sucker for sweets. It's also hard to deal with work and social functions where snacks and treats are set out for everyone."

Jeff knows it's tough for him to resist the siren song of a plate of cookies or bowl of chips, so he reserves a little room in his budget for treats. By tracking his calories diligently, keeping his meals to a set calorie limit, and avoiding "wasted" calorie expenditures, he's able to splurge a little on the things he loves most.

"Lose It! and calorie counting in general have drastically increased my awareness of how many calories various foods contain. Now I hesitate before having something like a bagel because I know I would rather 'spend' those calories on something else later in the day. I don't deprive myself of sweets. I just consume them in moderation now."

Reward yourself. The bagel tray will seem a lot less tempting when you know you have something much better waiting for you at home. Keep some treats in your house and make sure you leave room for them in your budget. Just make sure they are treats you can handle responsibly. Jeff and his wife have created a fun way of making sure neither of them binges on the treats they keep in the house.

"My wife and I do something we call 'Chocolate Genie,'" he says. "This means that I buy some treats that I love—let's say Reese's Peanut Butter Cups—and she hides the bag from me so I can't graze on them. And then, once a day, I can ask for my Chocolate Genie to come, which means that she goes to the stash that she has hidden, doles out an appropriate amount, and brings it to me. I do the same for her with her favorite treats."

The Chocolate Genie: Delivering Peanut Butter Cups and Weight Loss

Instead of Wasting Calories on Something Like	Jeff Skips It So He Can Save Room for	That Saves Him	If He Does That 5 Days a Week, That Equals	Over the Course of 10 Weeks, That Equals
Large bagel (350 calories)	Reese's Peanut Butter Cups, 1 package/2 cups (232 calories)	120 calories	600 calories	Almost 2 pounds

If eating treats in moderation is a challenge for you, it may not be a great idea to keep a bag of candy stashed in a drawer or a tub of ice cream in the freezer. Try purchasing your treats in single-serving sizes, such as 100-calorie snacks or other individually wrapped treats. Or buy only enough to last you through the week. If you know that eating an entire box of cookies on Monday means that you'll be treatless Tuesday through Friday, you'll be more likely to ration them.

Type #4: The Stress Eater

Inside all of us, there is a hormone that has the power to unleash our appetites like a monkey wrench opens a fire hydrant. This hormone is cortisol, the so-called stress hormone that's secreted when your body responds to prolonged periods of stress. When cortisol floods your body, it can set off cravings for the most calorie-rich, fattening, and carbohydrate-dense foods to be found within a 5-mile radius. And chances are that once you have your hands on them, you'll pig out like you've never seen food before.

But not everyone reacts to cortisol the same way. Some of us are more susceptible to its appetite-fueling effects than others. Do you find yourself looking for solace in a red velvet cupcake after a long, stressful day? Do you empty a bag of Doritos while your mother-in-law is in town? Order a pizza after looking at your credit card statement? If the answer to any of these questions is yes, then stress eating is a part of your life—and probably a major hindrance to your weight loss.

Here's another way to determine whether you're a stress-eating victim: Look at your weekly food logs. You probably tend to eat a lot of the same foods over and over again, but do you notice occasional calorie spikes that stand out from your usual activity? Can you remember the situations that prompted you to indulge in those foods? Chances are, if it wasn't a special occasion splurge, there was probably some serious stress involved.

If this is a behavior pattern you haven't taken seriously in the past, then today is the day to get it under control, because the science is clear: Not having a plan to cope with stress will continually push you into the Red Zone and undermine your progress.

Psychologists at the University of California, San Francisco, devised a study in which subjects were divided into groups and had to work together on challenging tasks. While the subjects were engaged in stressful activities, the scientists tempted them with an array of snacks: chocolate granola bars, potato chips, rice cakes, and pretzels. They found that the people who were most stressed-out by the tasks (as measured by their levels of cortisol) ate more than those who were less stressed, and they specifically sought out the most sugary, high-fat snacks available to them. Yup, cortisol is like a little gremlin in your stomach screaming for more, more, more—and it has a sweet tooth and a weakness for fat.

But there's another factor in the cortisol connection. What and how much you eat when cortisol is released in your body is determined by whether or not you've been depriving yourself before that. In another study in 2006, researchers gave men and women access to bowls of potato chips, M&M's, peanuts, and red grapes as they had them work on difficult anagrams. The most stressed-out women ate more M&M's than grapes, while the women who were the least stressed preferred the grapes. But the frazzled men didn't reach for the M&M's *or* the chips nearly as often as the stressed-out women did.

This surprising gender divide has a simple explanation: It's not that men are less susceptible to the effects of cortisol (or that they don't like chips and M&M's), it's that more of the women participating in the study were on a diet.

Studies show that people who are on diets are more likely than non-dieters to binge—and to keep binging once they give in to temptation. That is *especially* the case for dieters who feel they've been depriving themselves. Once a stressful situation leads to a giant bowl of ice cream, the floodgates open and all those weeks of repression cause you to indulge with a vengeance.

While cortisol is a pretty powerful force to be reckoned with, there are things you can do to put the gremlin back in its cage and keep your weight-loss progress moving right along. Here are a few strategies for taming stress eating.

Name that theme. Are there any common themes among your stress binges? Do they generally occur at work? Do they happen mostly in the evenings, when dealing with family, bills, or housework?

If you know there's a stressful situation or person that tends to push you over the edge, prepare yourself ahead of time for the stress that will inevitably come. Even the simple awareness of the fact that you're going into a situation that prompts you to overeat can help you brace for it and lower the risk that you'll give in. If your mom or a coworker always stresses you out, try using positive thinking. When that person says something characteristically irritating, don't say to yourself, "How could he say that to me?" Instead, try to think of it as, "Yep, that's George being George again." That kind of thinking can keep your stress levels down and stem the rising tide of cortisol from becoming a tsunami.

Understand your biology. Part of bracing for the event is thinking ahead about the outcome. Will giving in to stress and overeating make you feel any better once the ice cream container is empty and you're scraping away at that last smudge of cookie dough? Absolutely not. Ironically, it will only leave you feeling more stressed out. (And it'll give you a stomachache, to boot.) In fact, in a study published in the *British Journal of Psychiatry* in 2010, researchers showed—after tracking 3,500 men and women over 5 years—that a high consumption of processed foods increased the risk of developing depression, while people who ate healthier foods lowered their risk of developing the mood disorder.

The bottom line: Stress often leads to bingeing, and bingeing leads to more stress, more cortisol, and more weight gain. It's a vicious circle.

Smooth stress with lower-cal comfort food. Cortisol turns you into a fat-and-sugar-seeking missile. So forget about carrot sticks—you could eat a bag of them and still want a cheeseburger. Keep your desk at work and your pantry at home stocked with guilt-free substitutes that will satisfy your stress cravings. Or, when only that cheeseburger will do, be smart about it and order one that won't set you back too far.

Here are a few comfort food swaps that add up to big calorie savings.

Stress-Eating Substitutions

If You Like	Then Sub In	And Save	Do It 5 Times a Week and That Equals	After Only 10 Weeks, You've Dodged
Starbucks Double Chocolate Brownie (410 calories)	Clif Bar, Chocolate Brownie (240 calories)	170 calories	850 calories	2.5 pounds
Ruffles Original potato chips, 12 chips (160 calories)	American's Best Microwave popcorn, butter flavor, 2 cups popped (40 calories)	120 calories	600 calories	1.7 pounds
Starburst Fruit Chews, 8 pieces (160 calories)	Edy's No Sugar Added Fruit Bar, frozen (30 calories)	130 calories	650 calories	Almost 2 pounds

If You Like	Then Sub In	And Save	Do It 5 Times a Week and That Equals	After Only 10 Weeks, You've Dodged
Sbarro Pepperoni Pizza, 1 slice (730 calories)	Sbarro Cheese Pizza, 1 slice (460 calories)	270 calories	1,350 calories	Nearly 4 pounds
SuperSONIC Cheeseburger with ketchup (900 calories)	SONIC Cheeseburger with ketchup (630 calories)	270 calories	1,350 calories	Almost 4 pounds
SONIC Hamburger with ketchup (560 calories)	SONIC Corn Dog, 215 calories	345 calories	1,725 calories	4.9 pounds

Take your stress to the gym. Hands down, one of the best stress busters is exercise. Studies have repeatedly shown that adding a little movement to your life can improve mood, reduce anxiety and stress, and keep your calories in check. One 2010 study by researchers at the University of California, San Francisco, found that regular exercise even acts as a buffer against stress on a cellular level, keeping cortisol from ravaging your DNA. (In the study, sedentary people with highly stressful lives had greater signs of DNA damage than regular exercisers with equally stressful lives.)

But you don't even need a gym membership to reap the stress-busting benefits of exercise. All it takes is a walk around the block to ward off a cortisol-induced craving. In a study published in the journal *Appetite* in 2009, researchers took 25 people who regularly ate chocolate and made them abstain for 3 days. Then they exposed them to stress and gave them access to chocolate. They found that a brisk, 15-minute walk reduced their urges for chocolate, even when they inundated the subjects with ultradecadent images of chocolate.

A few other stress-busters that help neutralize the effects of cortisol include:

> Yoga

> Journaling (feelings, not food)

> Breathing exercises

> Peer support (talking to a supportive friend)

> Meditation

> Gardening

> Cleaning

> Adequate sleep (at least 7 hours each night)

> Massage

> Spending time with pets

Type #5: The Judger

Do you ever ask yourself why you're not losing weight when you feel like you're doing everything right?

You're not alone. We've all been inundated with so much junk food in healthy packaging that being a "health nut" these days can actually be bad for you—if you're not careful, that is. Food manufacturers are well aware that Americans are looking to lose weight, but those manufacturers need to keep up their profits somehow. Slapping healthy buzzwords on a package of high-calorie processed food is one way to do that.

Did you know that the so-called "all natural" chicken and turkey at your local supermarket may have been injected with salty broth, or that Minute Maid's "all natural" Berry Punch is loaded with high-calorie, high-fructose corn syrup? Even actual "healthy" foods—some of which offer many benefits—can be calorie budget destroyers if they're not eaten in moderation. Olive oil, avocados, nuts, whole grains, and even some fruits—these foods are high in nutrients and it's important that you eat them. But while dunking your bread in 2 tablespoons of olive oil will give you a nice dose of heart-healthy fats, you'll also be sopping up an additional 240 calories with your meal. You could spread 2 tablespoons of peanut butter on that bread and make it into a sandwich for fewer calories!

Here are some additional pointers to help you decode "healthy" food jargon.

They label, you decide. Why let the food manufacturers tell you what's good for you when you can just as easily look at nutrition labels and decide for yourself? Does a bottle of green tea with 8 teaspoons of sugar seem like a good idea to you? Of course not! So don't let Lipton fool you with its PureLeaf Green Tea with Honey. That's 120 calories worth of tea you'd be tossing back in one shot. Don't buy into marketing gimmicks. Read every food nutrition label and decide for yourself whether or not something makes sense for your calorie budget.

The good, the bad, and the unhealthy. Try not to categorize foods as "good" or "bad"—and definitely don't apply the same black-and-white thinking to your character. Eating an apple does not make you a "good" person any more than eating a cookie makes you a "bad" person!

It's easy to fall into the habit of eating unsatisfying "good" foods and then rewarding yourself with "bad" ones—quickly undoing any progress that you've made. Plus, foods that seem like "good" choices are often even worse, calorie wise, than those "bad" foods you're avoiding. So take the virtue and sin out of food, and know that sometimes a butter croissant will do more for your weight-loss efforts than a high-fiber apple bran muffin.

A Healthy Dose of Reality

Instead of "Being Good" and Ordering This	Get What You Really Want	And Save	Do That 3 Times a Week and Save	Over 10 Weeks, That Equals
Ruby Tuesday Avocado Turkey Burger (1,130 calories)	Ruby Tuesday Ruby's Classic Burger (1,091 calories)	39 calories	117 calories	About 0.3 pound
McDonald's Filet-O-Fish (380 calories)	McDonald's Cheeseburger (300 calories)	80 calories	240 calories	Almost 0.7 pound
Starbucks Apple Bran Muffin (350 calories)	Starbucks Butter Croissant (310 calories)	40 calories	120 calories	About 0.3 pound
Applebee's Apple Walnut Chicken Salad (1,000 calories)	Applebee's Bacon Cheddar Cheeseburger (940 calories)	60 calories	180 calories	0.5 pound
Subway 6" Tuna sandwich (530 calories)	Subway 6" Steak & Cheese sandwich (380 calories)	150 calories	450 calories	Almost 1.5 pounds

If you're an eco-conscious eater, "good" and "bad" have other connotations for you. While your efforts to green our planet are applause-worthy, don't forget that words like "organic," "sustainable," and "grass-fed" do not necessarily mean "low in calories." Being good to the Earth doesn't automatically mean you're making good choices for your waistline.

Calories over quantity. If eating larger portions of lower-calorie foods is your thing, that's fine. But be aware that some foods can throw you off your budget when you indulge with too much abandon. For example, almonds are often touted for their nutritional power—and they certainly are a high-protein snack that delivers a nice dose of vitamin E and mono-unsaturated fats. But if you eat just ½ cup of almonds (easy to do in one sitting), you're taking in 400 calories. A serving of almonds is actually only about 20 nuts (140 calories). When eating calorie-dense foods like nuts or dried fruits, portion control is essential.

Even some fruits, if eaten in excess, can add up to lots of extra calories—especially if they're packed in syrup, frozen with added sugar, or dried and sprinkled with sugar. If you like snacking on fruit, keep in mind that not all fruits are created equal in terms of calories: high-water fruits like cantaloupe, watermelon, and berries are very low in calories, while bananas, cherries, and other high-sugar fruits pack more calories. Portion size also matters, and a lot more than you might think. Remember that for most fruits, like strawberries, grapes, berries, and melons, one serving is $\frac{1}{2}$ cup. It's fine to eat more than that, just as long as you're recording each serving you ate in your log.

The chart below shows you just how essential portion size is when it comes to fruit. When you choose fruits that are less calorie-dense, you can eat a much bigger serving for fewer calories.

Make Progress in the Produce Aisle

For the Calorie Cost of This	You Can Have All of This
Banana (121 calories)	Cantaloupe, $\frac{1}{2}$ of an entire melon (100 calories)
Del Monte Fruit Naturals Pineapple Chunks, 1 cup (140 calories)	Diced watermelon, 3 cups (120 calories)
Fresh cherries, 2 cups (180 calories)	Fresh blueberries, 3 cups (190 calories)
Dried apple rings, 8 pieces (120 calories)	Small apples, 2 (110 calories)
Mango, large (150 calories)	Diced honeydew, 2 cups or about 40 pieces (122 calories)
Raisins, 1 small box/1.5 oz (129 calories)	Red grapes, 2 cups (124 calories)

Personalizing Weight Loss

This is where your Lose It! experience gets about as personal as it can be. Now it's up to you to look over your data and study yourself. Your food log is more than just a record of what you've eaten. It's also a written record of your priorities and behavior—one that will help you diagnose the motives that underscore your everyday choices.

Even a cursory look at your data from the past week or month will reveal some surprising patterns—the fact that you're getting a scary amount of calories from beverages, for example, or that it's a bad idea to have a tub of ice cream in the freezer on a Sunday night (especially without any alternatives to fall back on if a stress-related food craving strikes). Like Charles, you may even find that the biggest barrier to achieving your target weight is a single, 2-minute window of time that occurs every day, when you're face-to-face with your greatest sugary temptation.

No matter what your vices may be, once you discern your own blind spots, you can adjust your strategy accordingly for the road ahead.

Chapter Six

Stuck in Neutral

Push Through Plateaus and Setbacks

What happened?

You were doing so well—tracking your meals, racking up negative calories, and steering clear of the Red Zone. You were seeing and feeling results: lost pounds, increased energy, improved health. And then, suddenly, the downward slope of weight loss became as flat as, well, a pancake.

Plateaus are like exes: Everyone has one, and we all get over them eventually. This is the point where most diets fail, and it can definitely be tempting to throw in the towel when you're not seeing the results you've become used to. There will be frustration. There will be disappointment, anger, and maybe even a few tears. But once you get past the shock of your first major setback, you'll be better for it.

That's right: Plateaus can be positive. Just like any stumbling block in life, they offer a chance for growth. Plateaus are an opportunity to reassess your game plan, figure out what's working and what's not, and shake up your routine.

WEIGHT IS JUST A NUMBER

The number on your bathroom scale might seem like it's glued in place, but there's more to losing weight than the number on the scale. Even though it's gratifying to watch that number fall further and further, pounds lost aren't the only way to measure your success.

Another gauge of your efforts is your body composition—that is, the ratio of fat to muscle in your body. The more you work out and lose weight, the more lean muscle mass you add to your frame, and the more fat you burn.

Body composition is important for a couple of reasons. First, having a leaner body promotes long-term health. In fact, a study by the Mayo Clinic in 2008 found that body fat percentage was a much better predictor of heart disease risk than either obesity or body mass index (BMI). Second, having a leaner body also helps your weight-loss efforts. A pound of fat burns around 2 calories a day to maintain itself, but a pound of muscle—at rest—burns *triple* that amount.

Health authorities recommend that men maintain a body-fat percentage below 25 percent and women maintain body-fat percentage below 31 percent. There are several ways to measure your body composition; some of the most accurate tests are available through your doctor. But there are two cheap, easy ways to get a rough estimate at home. The first is to purchase a pair of inexpensive Accu-Measure Body Fat Calipers (available online for less than $10), which will give you a good sense of your body fat percentage. But the second, simpler way to determine whether your body is getting leaner is to ask yourself the following questions: Do your clothes feel looser? Have you lost inches off of your arms, legs, and waist? Do you find yourself tightening your belt another notch? Are you noticing signs of muscle tone and definition that you haven't seen in ages (or maybe ever)?

If your bathroom scale seems to be frozen in time but your body is getting leaner, then you *haven't* hit a plateau—you're just adding more muscle to your frame. And because muscle weighs more than fat, you may not be seeing results on the scale at the moment, but if you keep doing what you've been doing, you'll see that number budge in a week or two.

If, on the other hand, your clothes still feel snug and you're not noticing any more muscle tone, then you may in fact have hit a true plateau. In that case, you need a plan of action for busting through it.

HOW DID IT COME TO THIS?
FINDING THE CAUSE OF YOUR PLATEAU

In order to overcome your plateau, you first have to diagnose it. It's time to take a step back, look at the data that you've generated through logging your food, and be prepared to make a few changes to your daily routine.

Everybody hits plateaus for different reasons, but after analyzing the data of 10,000 Lose It! users, some clear patterns emerge. In this chapter, you'll discover some of the most common pitfalls that lead to plateaus and the quickest and most efficient strategies for getting back on track.

Pitfall #1: Bugs (in Your Tracking)

What if you're doing everything right? You're evaluating calorie counts, logging your meals, steering clear of the Red Zone—but you're not losing weight. How can that be possible?

When you hit a plateau, your first order of business is to look for bugs in the system. Even if you are 100 percent diligent about recording your numbers, there's a chance that your numbers may not be accurate. Did you know that some of the nutritional information listed on packaged foods and restaurant menus is wrong? A study conducted by scientists at Tufts University and published in the *Journal of the American Dietetic Association* in 2010 found that fast-food meals—especially those advertised as healthier, low-calorie options—contained an average of *18 percent more calories* than the figures listed in their nutritional information.

"Some individual restaurant items contained up to 200 percent of stated values," the scientists wrote. But that's not all: The same team at Tufts found that many packaged foods contained more calories than the amount listed on their labels. That's because the FDA allows manufacturers a pretty large margin of error: an average of 8 percent! In other words, that bag of Doritos you bought the other day may have had more calories than the label indicated.

If you're not concerned about your weight, then hey, the more free

AN EXTRA 20 PERCENT: NO BIGGIE, RIGHT?

Let's say you ate ½ cup—one serving—of Ben & Jerry's Cheesecake Brownie ice cream four times a week and logged that it contained 250 calories each time. But what if it really contained 295 calories per serving?

After 1 month = 720 extra calories = 0.2 pound gained

After 6 months = 4,320 extra calories = 1.2 pounds gained

After 1 year = 8,640 extra calories = 2.5 pounds gained

food the better! But by now you realize that when you're tracking calories, eating a frozen dinner that you *think* contains 400 calories but that really contains 440 can be a big problem, especially if you're eating it on a regular basis.

So how do you know when you're being overserved?

Weigh it yourself. Invest in a kitchen scale—you can find reliable digital models for less than $20 at Wal-Mart. If you buy a bag of Doritos that lists 50 grams of food on the label but you weigh it and get a reading of 60 grams, then you'll know you've got a bag with 300 calories in it, not 250. That doesn't mean you can't eat all of the chips, it just means that you have to log them accurately.

Many Lose It! users keep scales on their kitchen countertops for convenience and precision, whether they're weighing packaged foods or measuring out pasta and cheese for home recipes. Jennifer Mueller Krause of Washington says, "I use a kitchen scale to know exactly what I'm eating. There's no guesswork: It tells you the exact amount!"

Be wary of side dishes. The regular burger patties at McDonald's are about as cookie-cutter as the golden arches outside—they don't vary too drastically from one patty to the next. But a side of fries has a lot more variables—one day your "small fry" order might fit perfectly into the container and another day it may overflow into the bag. At Boston Market, a side of mashed potatoes might fill the entire container on Monday and be half that size on Tuesday. At most fast-food joints, side dishes are a giant question mark, from a calorie standpoint. In fact, the Tufts University team found that side dishes can increase the calorie content of an entire meal by 245 percent more than what's stated in the restaurant's nutritional information.

When you order a side dish, make sure it's not a "super side." If you frequent a place that you know tends to be overly generous with its serving sizes, don't be shy about asking your server for the proper portion.

Know your margin of error. We know that the restaurants and food manufacturers have a margin of error when it comes to calorie counts, but what's *your* margin of error? You might think your portion sizes and servings are exactly the same as they were back when you started logging, but are you sure?

Your ability to identify normal portion sizes can degrade over time, and people tend to underestimate their portion sizes when they use large bowls, plates, and silverware. One study in 2003 found that nutritionists, of all people, overserved themselves by 31 percent when they were given large bowls and by 15 percent when they were given large spoons.

When you pour a normal serving of food into a big bowl, your brain sees the empty space and tells you to fill it up. So avoid eating from oversize plates and silverware at restaurants whenever possible, and if your plates at home are oversize, use salad plates for your everyday meals.

It's also a good idea to give yourself a refresher course in portion sizes by breaking out the measuring cups if you haven't been using them for a while. If your "eyeballed" portions have been gradually increasing, chances are that's why the number on your scale has been staying put.

Pitfall #2: Not Eating Enough

Okay, you've double-checked your portion sizes and haven't found any problems. You've been staying clear of the Red Zone and tracking every last bite: You're definitely not eating too much. Could it be possible that you're not eating *enough?*

Actually, yes—it's quite possible. Like any machine, your body needs fuel to function properly. When it doesn't get enough fuel and it's essentially running on empty, it conserves the energy it does have. And one of the ways it does this is by slowing down your metabolism so you burn through your remaining fuel at a slower pace.

As you learned in Chapter 1, your body weight is one of the factors that determines your metabolism. The less you weigh, the lower your metabolic rate. So as you slim down, that rate slows significantly and your body burns a lot fewer calories than it was burning when you started your journey. Combine a slower metabolism with too few calories and you've got a recipe for a plateau.

So ask yourself this: Are you taking in enough calories to kick-start your metabolism?

While the Lose It! program guidelines suggest that you lose no more than 2 pounds a week, many people who want to lose more weight at a faster pace deliberately create daily calorie budgets that are 200, 300, or even 400 calories less than the suggested budget. Drastically reducing calorie intake will certainly help you lose more weight at first, but eventually, if your body isn't getting an adequate supply of calories, your metabolic fire will start to wane and your weight loss will flatten out. If you exercise regularly, you have an even greater risk of hitting this plateau. Without enough calories, you'll have less energy and your workouts will suffer. You can only run so far or lift so much weight without any fuel in your tank.

All things being equal, a person who eats just up to the Red Line is likely to burn more calories during exercise than someone who skips meals and hits the gym on an empty stomach.

If you're consistently coming in 200 calories underbudget, then try eating right up to the Red Line over the course of at least 3 days. If you're coming in 300 calories underbudget every day, then add at least a couple hundred calories a day for 3 to 7 days. You'll still be finishing in the Green Zone, so you *will* lose weight, but you'll be surprised by how quickly the weight starts to disappear again. That's exactly what happened to Lose It! user Mark Castlebury of Virginia.

"I used to short myself 200 or 300 calories a day, and when I did that I would hold onto the weight. But when I started eating up to the line, I actually shed more weight!" he says. Mark has lost more than 40 pounds using Lose It! He found that the more he exercised, the more

TIPS AND TRICKS:
ADJUSTING YOUR CALORIE BUDGET

If you think your budget may be a little high, there's a simple way to tweak it in four easy steps. Start by pulling up the app and looking at the home screen.

1. At the bottom of the screen, click on the tab that says "Goals."

2. About halfway up the screen, you should see a tab that says "Modify Program." Click on it.

3. At the bottom of the next screen, you'll see a tab that says "Daily Calorie Budget." Click on it.

4. Finally, click on the tab for "Adjustment." That'll bring you to a screen where you can add or subtract calories from your overall budget. We recommend that you don't go overboard. Try starting off with a small change, no more than about 5 percent. See how that feels for 10 days before making any additional tweaks.

calories he needed to eat to keep his metabolism going and to fuel his workouts. "It's like you have to fuel your body for it to lose weight. You need to stoke yourself. To do more, you have to give it more, and then it burns more."

"I figured out," he added, "that if I tried to give myself an extra cushion by not eating up to the line, then my body would go into starvation mode and I wouldn't lose as much weight."

Sometimes all it takes is one weekend. Sabrina Euton of Atlanta hit a frustrating plateau after losing nearly 30 pounds. She'd been consistently coming in under her calorie budget, so she decided to take advantage of an upcoming holiday and splurge a little in hopes that it would get her out of her rut.

"I kind of got stuck at 27 pounds lost, and for about a week, I didn't lose any weight," she said. "So I took a couple days off for St. Patrick's Day. It was a little bit of a shock to my body, but at the same time, I got over my plateau!"

Pitfall #3: Getting Stuck In a Rut

Anything can grow boring and stale if you do it long enough. The human body is expert at adaptation. It craves homeostasis and will fight to adjust to any food or exercise that comes its way. Unfortunately, too much adjustment can quickly result in too little weight loss.

But adding some variety to your diet and workouts can be energizing, and it might allow you to discover some new strategies that work even better than your tried-and-true favorites.

If you've been eating the same foods day in, day out, it's definitely time to add a little flavor to your life. Go online and download some new recipes. Ask other Lose It! users for their favorite healthy eating tips. Buy new foods at the grocery store, change your order at your favorite take-out place, and experiment with new restaurants.

Then take a look at the breakdown of carbs, protein, and fat in your diet. Your calorie intake will always be the most important piece of this puzzle, but when you're trying to shake those last few pounds that just won't budge, experimenting with a new combination of daily macronutrients could be the little push that gets you past the final 5- or 10-pound tipping point. Some people find that adding more protein and dialing back on the carbs—even by as little as 10 percent—helps rev up their weight loss again, while others find that keeping their protein intake steady and beefing up their intake of healthy fats and complex carbs makes the difference. Your body may be missing something, and shifting the ratio of carbs, fat, and protein might give it exactly what it needs to bust through that plateau.

If you adjust your carbs or protein by 10 percent and the scale registers a change in the right direction, then bump that change up to 20 percent and see if the weight loss continues.

WHY VARIETY MATTERS

Once you've added some variety to your eating routine, it's time to look at the next piece of the plateau puzzle: your exercise habits. Are you still exercising as much as you were 3 months ago? More important, are you exercising with the same intensity?

If your runs are getting shorter and slower and your gym sessions are becoming briefer and less frequent, it's no wonder your waistline is in limbo.

Bust Through Your Plateau with Higher-Protein Snacks

Replace This	With This	The Result
Yoplait Yogurt, Low Fat French Vanilla I serving 170 calories 5 g protein 33 g carbs	Light n' Lively Lowfat Cottage Cheese I serving 80 calories 12 g protein 6 g carbs	You'll cut 90 calories and 27 g carbs and gain 7 g protein.
Quaker Oatmeal Squares Cereal I cup 210 calories 6 g protein 44 g carbs	Quaker Instant Oatmeal, Original 2 packets 200 calories 8 g protein 38 g carbs	You'll cut 10 calories and 6 g carbs and gain 2 g protein.
Lay's potato chips I serving 150 calories 2 g protein 15 g carbs	Beef jerky I large piece 82 calories 7 g protein 2 g carbs	You'll cut 68 calories and 13 g carbs and gain 5 g protein.
Power Bar Performance, Chocolate I bar 240 calories 8 g protein 45 g carbs	Oh Yeah! Bar, Vanilla Toffee Fudge I bar 190 calories 15 g protein 17 g carbs	You'll cut 50 calories and 28 g carbs and gain 7 g protein.
Peanut M&M's I package (1.74 oz) 250 calories 5 g protein 30 g carbs	Planters Trail Mix, Mixed Nuts & Raisins I serving 150 calories 5 g protein 10 g carbs	You'll cut 100 calories and 20 g carbs.

Even if you're burning just 50 fewer calories a day, that can be enough to keep your weight static.

Not only is it important to keep up the intensity and duration of your workouts, it's also essential to keep changing your routine. Running the same route, in the same park, at the same pace, for the same distance—to the point where you could practically run it in your sleep—may be your favorite thing. But after a while your body gets used to this workout, and if you're not challenging your body, your muscles won't be stimulated in the same way that they were when you first started running that route. When your body becomes accustomed to your exercise routine, it becomes more efficient at it, so you end up burning fewer calories. In fact, a 2009 study in the *International Journal of Obesity* found that runners who didn't increase the mileage and intensity of their runs over time gained more weight than those who did.

As you lose weight and get fitter, maintaining intensity requires more exercise. Your new, sleeker, lighter frame won't respond in the same way

If you decided to be a little less active every day, what would the long-term effects look like? You might be surprised by how much weight you gain when you burn just 50 calories less a day.

1 week = 350 calories = 0.1 pound

1 month = 1,500 calories = just under 0.5 pound

2 months = 3,000 calories = more than 0.9 pound

3 months = 4,500 calories = about 1.3 pounds

1 year = about 18,000 calories = a little more than 5 pounds

Amp Up Your Workout to Burn More Calories

If You Do This	Add This	You'll Burn an Extra	Do It 3 Times a Week to Burn	Over 10 Weeks That Equals an Extra
Weight training, 1 hour (385 calories)	Plyometrics. Add a set of jumps after each set.	130 calories each workout	400 additional calories	1.2 pounds
Walking at 3 mph, 1 hour (206 calories)	Swing your arms when you walk, pumping them with each step.	30 calories each workout	90 additional calories	0.3 pound
Power walking at 3.5 mph, 1 hour (240 calories)	Wear a weighted vest or carry light dumbbells in each hand.	45 calories each workout	135 additional calories	Nearly 0.5 pound
Exercising without stretching first	Before every workout, do some mild stretching for 15 minutes.	43 calories each workout	132 additional calories	Nearly 0.5 pound
Running on the treadmill at 6 mph, 1 hour (650 calories)	Alternate between flat and a 3.5 percent incline every 5 to 10 minutes.	80 calories each workout	240 additional calories	Nearly 0.75 pound

*All information in this chart is based on a 160-pound person. The number of calories you burn will vary depending on your weight.

to your old exercises—you won't burn as many calories because the same run at the same old pace won't be as tough for you. If you've lost weight but haven't stepped up your pace, then it's time to refer back to the estimates of intensity in the exercise chapter (see page 84). You need to switch into a higher gear.

It doesn't matter if you're climbing stairs or cycling on a stationary bike—when your routine goes stale, your body adapts and your bottom line suffers. Your exercise routine needs the occasional element of surprise to keep your body guessing—and losing. So try squashing the status quo with new routines and challenges that stimulate different muscle groups and force your body to work harder.

If you like running or biking long distances, then try the high-intensity interval workouts on page 76. If you're already a high-intensity devotee, then try some longer-duration cardio that will help improve your endurance. If you're only doing cardio, then start doing some resistance training, which will add metabolically active muscle and help you burn more calories at rest.

Mix It Up

The name of the game is variety. Jazzing up your gym routine helps you psychologically, as well, by giving you the motivation and the mental boost you need in order to keep exercising. Simply put, variety leads to enjoyment, and enjoyment leads to *adherence.* One study by researchers at the University of Florida at Gainesville in 2001 found that people who repeated the same aerobic exercises over an 8-week period were far more likely to quit their cardio routines than those who spiced things up. In the study, people were split into three groups—one that was encouraged to vary their exercise, another that performed the same exercise every time, and one that was given no instructions. Of the 52 people who eventually

Shake Up Your Routine

If You're Doing This	Then Mix Things Up with This	You'll Burn an Extra	Do It 3 Times a Week to Burn	Over 2 Months That Equals
Jogging at 5 mph, 30 minutes (290 calories)	Running up stairs at high intensity, 30 minutes (525 calories)	235 calories	705 additional calories	Almost 2 pounds
Cycling on a stationary bike at moderate intensity, 30 minutes (247 calories)	Jumping rope at moderate intensity, 30 minutes (302 calories)	55 calories	165 additional calories	Almost 0.5 pound
Walking at 2 mph, 30 minutes (91 calories)	Low-impact aerobics, 30 minutes (183 calories)	92 calories	276 additional calories	Almost 0.75 pound
Yoga, 30 minutes (88 calories)	Vinyasa yoga, a more intense form than regular yoga, 30 minutes (223 calories)	135 calories	405 additional calories	About 1 pound
Elliptical machine at moderate intensity, 30 minutes (150 calories)	Treadmill, 12-minute miles, 30 minutes (264 calories)	114 calories	342 additional calories	0.8 pound

*All information in this chart is based on a 160-pound person. The number of calories you burn will vary depending on your weight.

dropped out, the majority were in the nonvarying group. The participants who engaged in a variety of exercises were more likely to exercise consistently, and they reported higher rates of enjoyment than the exercisers in the other groups.

So the moral is, don't allow the ease of your routine to force you into a mental rut. Mix it up to stay motivated.

For example, if you're a treadmill junkie, try signing up for a spinning class to get your heart pumping. If you're starting to feel like a caged hamster on the elliptical machine, why not go for a long bike ride in the park or a swim at the beach? If you're lifting the same weight over and over again with diminishing results, try a more rigorous program, such as P90X (a combination of strength training, cardio, yoga, plyometrics, and stretching). Or try a martial arts class for a new challenge that'll still build muscle and endurance while also exterminating calories.

Pitfall #4: You Sleep What You Sow

At first glance, it might be hard to see how sleep and weight loss could possibly be connected. But years of research have shown that adequate sleep is essential to weight loss, and a habit of burning the midnight oil could be pushing you to plateau.

That's right: Sabotaging your sleep cycle will almost always sabotage your weight loss. Your body needs plenty of rest in order to properly produce the hormones that regulate your appetite: ghrelin, which prompts you to feel hungry, and leptin, the hormone that lets you know when you're full. When you don't get enough sleep, you throw this delicate system out of whack.

A study published in the *American Journal of Clinical Nutrition* showed that people ended up eating more than 500 extra calories on days when they'd only gotten 4 hours of sleep the previous night, compared to days when they'd gotten 8 hours of sleep. That's roughly 22 percent more calories! And a 2009 University of Chicago study had similar findings: Subjects took in significantly more calories from snacks and carbs when operating on $5\frac{1}{2}$ hours of sleep than they did on $8\frac{1}{2}$ hours of rest.

Being sleep-deprived seems to send a message to your brain: "Hey, since we're up and awake a lot longer, we need more fuel!" So your body starts spewing out more ghrelin and suppressing leptin, putting you in a near-constant state of hunger. It's a one-two punch that can halt your weight loss. If you've hit a plateau and you think lack of sleep might be your problem, ask yourself the following:

> Do you consistently wake up feeling groggy and exhausted?

> Do you feel irritable or sleepy during the day?

> Do you ever fall asleep or feel your eyelids getting heavy while driving?

> Do you need a steady supply of caffeine to get through the day?

> Do other people often tell you that you look tired?

> Do you often have trouble concentrating?

> Do you have trouble staying awake when you sit still for more than a few minutes?

If you answered yes to three or more of these questions, then you may very well be sleep-deprived. A typical night's rest should be somewhere in the range of 7 to 8 hours. Anything less, and you run the risk of seeing the readings on your scale flatline.

You're working so hard to keep the weight off during the day, it would be a shame to let a couple hours of lost sleep at night ruin your progress. Plan to get at least 7 hours of shut-eye every night. If you have problems falling asleep or staying asleep, you may find the following strategies helpful.

> Keep your room dark during sleep hours—no glowing computer screens or open shades. Wear a sleep mask, if you need to.

> Lower the temperature in your bedroom. Studies have found that the optimal temperature for sleep is between 60° and 68°F.

> Shut off the TV at least an hour before bed. The flickering light can interfere with your body clock, and television can be noisy and overstimulating.

> Don't exercise before bed. Working out during the day can help you fall asleep faster at night, but if you exercise too close to bedtime, the adrenaline and other hormones still coursing through your veins will keep you wide awake and staring up at the ceiling. As a general rule, try to avoid intense physical activity in the 3 hours before you plan on going to bed.

> Try a relaxation technique. Shut your eyes and slowly inhale through your nose, counting to five in your mind. Exhale slowly, counting to eight in your mind as you expel the air from your lungs. Repeat at least four times.

Pitfall #5: Water Weight

Do you feel puffy and bloated on a regular basis? Do you ever feel like you're sporting a paunch that you just can't shake, no matter how much you weigh?

Struggling with water weight is common during weight loss. The solution seems pretty simple: If your body's holding onto extra water, you should drink less water, right? Wrong. What many people think of as a problem caused by excess water is really a problem of not enough water. If you've been exercising regularly and not drinking enough water, then your body will do everything it can to hold onto every drop of this life-sustaining liquid. That's also the case if you've been traveling, eating a lot of salty foods (think processed foods, canned soups, and restaurant meals), or drinking too much alcohol or caffeine. When your body isn't getting enough water, it won't release the little that it has.

There are two clues that can help you determine whether you're properly hydrated: your level of thirst and the color of your urine. If you feel parched or thirsty at all, then you're probably already a little dehydrated. And if your urine is any darker than straw-color, you're also in need of water.

If you're physically active, routinely sipping water is a must. Drink the equivalent of at least two to three 12-ounce bottles of water a day, along with your other usual beverages.

Don't worry about the "eight glasses of water a day" rule. Studies show it's a myth. We do need plenty of water, but according to the Institute of Medicine of the National Academies, you can meet your body's need for liquids in many ways, including by drinking tea, coffee (as long as you're not drinking more than two or three cups a day), and juice (as long as you're counting those calories), as well as by eating fruits and vegetables that have a higher water content.

And don't worry about the extra water you're drinking leading to water weight. In a study published in the *Journal of the American College of Nutrition* in 2000, scientists found that properly hydrating with water and other beverages actually resulted in "slight body weight loss."

Pitfall #6: Forgetting That Every Calorie Counts

At the end of the day, you're ultimately going to get over a plateau in the same way that you've been losing weight all along—with small calorie deficits that add up to that all-important 3,500-calorie mark. Keep thinking of little ways that you can eliminate small blocks of calories here and there. Do you sneak in little tastes while cooking dinner? Steal a few fries from your kid's plate? Are there any more calories you can easily skim—say, the tablespoon of honey you add to your tea or the jam and butter you spread on your toast? What about that bottle of Gatorade you chug after every workout?

See a few more ideas for cutting calories to help you push your way past a plateau on the opposite page.

SOMETIMES A PLATEAU ISN'T A PLATEAU

Whether this is your first plateau or your fifth, there's always a chance you'll run into another one somewhere down the line, especially as you get closer and closer to your target weight. The less you weigh, the harder it is to lose pounds.

But if you get within 5 or 10 pounds of your target weight and those last few pounds just won't budge, your body may be trying to tell you something: It doesn't need to lose any more weight. The weight-loss goal you set for yourself months ago may not be realistic for your body type or your lifestyle.

Plateau-Busting Food Swaps

If You Hit a Plateau While Eating This	Then Try This	Do It 4 Times a Week and Save	Over 10 Weeks, That Equals
Starbucks Caffè Latte, made with skim milk, 8 oz (110 calories)	Regular coffee with 3 Tbsp fat-free milk (17 calories)	372 calories	1 pound
Häagen-Dazs Dulce De Leche ice cream, ½ cup (290 calories)	Skinny Cow Caramel & Vanilla Bar (100 calories)	760 calories	More than 2 pounds
IHOP Belgian Waffle, 1 (390 calories)	Van's Gourmet Belgian Waffle, 7-Grain, 1 (115 calories)	1,100 calories	More than 3 pounds
Subway Peanut Butter Cookies, 2 (440 calories)	Nabisco Nutter Butter 100 Calorie Granola Bars, 2 (200 calories)	960 calories	Almost 3 pounds
Ritz Crackers, 5, with Kraft Mild Cheddar Cheese, 2 oz (320 calories)	Ritz Whole Wheat Crackers, 5, with Athenos Reduced Fat Feta Cheese, 1 oz (130 calories)	760 calories	More than 2 pounds
Golden Grahams cereal, 1 cup, with whole milk, ½ cup (235 calories)	Large graham cracker squares, 2, with peanut butter, 1 tsp (100 calories)	540 calories	1. 5 pounds
Baked potato, 1 large, with Tostitos Salsa and Breakstone's Sour Cream, 2 Tbsp each (355 calories)	Baked potato, small, with Amy's Organic Salsa and Breakstone's Fat-Free Sour Cream, 2 Tbsp each (170 calories)	740 calories	More than 2 pounds

There are achievements that are even more important than the number you see on the scale. Are you lean and fit? Do you have more energy and stamina? Are you wearing a smaller size? Is your blood pressure normal, your cholesterol at a good level? Is your doctor happy with your weight loss?

If the answer to these questions is yes, then try not to obsess over a few pounds. It's important to recognize and take pride in your accomplishments. You've changed your life for the better; in all likelihood, you've extended it by a few years, as well. So start enjoying your new life in your new body, and pat yourself on the back for a job well done.

But don't close the book just yet. You're ready for the final chapter of your transformation. Now that the weight is off, you've got to protect the fruits of your labor. Maintaining weight loss involves less work than you've done up to this point, but it's not without its challenges. You've invested too much to gain the weight back at this point.

It's time to master maintenance mode.

Chapter Seven

Lose It for Life

Create Your Maintenance Plan

As you know by now, losing weight is all about numbers—the number of calories you're putting away versus the number of calories you're putting to use. That's one fundamental law of human biology that you simply can't ignore.

Once you lose the weight, there's another project to tackle: keeping it off. And what a project it is. The statistics on weight maintenance are sobering: According to a nationwide study conducted by the Centers for Disease Control and Prevention (CDC) in 2007, 33 percent of people who lose a "substantial" amount of weight regain some or all of those dropped pounds within a year. That's one in three people, and by some accounts, that's a conservative estimate. In fact, many obesity researchers say the number of dieters who eventually regain all or most of the weight they've lost, whether it's a year later or a decade later, is more than *double* that figure.

These numbers paint a somewhat bleak picture and underscore what anyone who's ever been on a diet knows to be true: Keeping the weight off is no easy task. But the good news is, the statistics we have for weight maintenance largely reflect the experiences of Americans who have lost weight on 30-day plans and other extreme diets that include methods that just aren't sustainable. If you've been slimming down with Lose It!, then you already know that diets simply don't work. True weight loss can only occur when you change your lifestyle and make smarter, more economical decisions about what you eat. You need to strike a balance between eating what you love and making choices that support your long-term health.

So if you've achieved your weight-loss goal, what now? The decision you make today may very well be the most important one of your entire weight-loss journey. It's one that could result in lifelong weight maintenance or an endless cycle of weight gain and loss.

MAINTENANCE MODE: WATCH YOUR BUDGET MAGICALLY GROW

Now that the extra weight is gone, you might feel tempted to stop logging. After all, you've got this weight-loss thing down, right? You've trained yourself to think economically about food, and like most Lose It! users, by the time you reach your goal, you can rattle off the calorie counts in your usual foods with precision. Even still, it's a good idea to continue tracking, at least for a few weeks.

Here's why.

On the day you reach your goal, your personalized Lose It! plan automatically switches into Maintenance Mode. Since you're no longer in the process of losing weight, this means that your calorie budget will grow. The app will make the adjustment automatically. If you're counting calories manually, it's simple to do this yourself: Just take the amount of weight you were

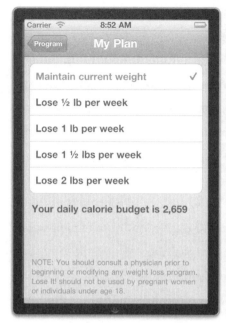

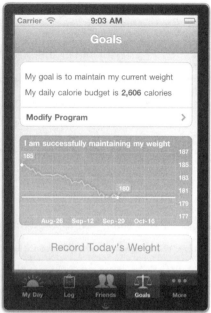

Once you reach your target weight, your plan will automatically switch to maintenance mode. Your daily budget will increase just enough to keep you at your new weight.

losing each week and add that amount of calories to your weekly budget. If you were losing weight at a rate of 1 pound a week, then your weekly budget will grow by 3,500 calories (the number of calories in 1 pound, since you're no longer trying to lose that pound). That's the equivalent of 500 additional calories each day. If you had the app set so you'd lose 2 pounds a week, then your budget will grow by 7,000 calories a week (2 × 3,500 calories). That's an extra 1,000 calories a day!

That's quite a lot of extra room.

If you were losing 2 pounds a week on a budget of 1,800 calories a day, for example, then your budget would make a dramatic leap to 2,800 calories a day. No matter what number you end up with, you may find that you don't need all of the extra calories. In fact, many people in maintenance mode say they end up with far more daily calories than they could ever consume.

It sounds like a good problem to have, and to some extent, it is. You end up with a large buffer zone. But it's critical that you exercise some caution. Remember, you didn't become overweight in a day; it took years of overeating. You didn't wake up one day and decide to start eating double the amount of food you were eating the day before. Incorporating more and more food and larger and larger meals into your life was a gradual process.

Dropping the weight with Lose It! was also a gradual process. You reached your goal in small increments, 100 calories at a time. It's important to be aware of the fact that it's easy to gain back the weight in the same way, with small changes that add up: skipping workouts here and there, spending a few more hours on the couch each week, eating a nightly bowl of ice cream that swells from one scoop to three.

Just ask Brad Weston, 37, of Georgia. Brad lost more than 70 pounds with Lose It! and has kept it off for more than a year.

Brad was a self-described "fat kid" who turned into a fat adult. After trying a few diet plans over the years and finding them completely unsustainable, Lose It!, he says, was a godsend.

"It became kind of fun. That sounds a little weird, but every day there was a sense of accomplishment. Instead of saying, 'Hey, I want to lose 30 pounds,' you know that each day—so long as that number doesn't stay red each day has its own individual victory. I liked the daily accountability. Every day you know exactly where you are at any given time and can plan accordingly."

But after reaching his target weight, Brad quit tracking his foods and, for a while at least, he all but forgot about all the hard work that had gotten him to his goal.

"I just kind of stopped using it," he said.

Brad kept exercising, thinking it would be enough to counteract all of the extra food he was enjoying. It wasn't. Without the program by his side, there was no way of tracking the calories coming in and the calories going out. Then one day Brad stepped on a scale and discovered, to his amazement, that he had regained 10 pounds. Somewhere along the way he'd made a wrong turn that set him on a dangerous path, and his success was starting to slip away.

Brad was lucky he caught those 10 pounds before they turned into

RED FLAGS

Gaining weight? Your scale will tell the tale. But there are other benchmarks you can use to gauge your progress, as well.

1. Are you able to easily button your favorite pair of jeans, or do you find that they fit a little more snugly than they did a few weeks ago?

2. Is the band of your wristwatch feeling tighter?

3. When you put on your belt, do you find yourself reaching for a new belt hole—one that provides a little more room?

4. Is your normally comfortable bra suddenly digging into your back?

5. If you're a stress eater, do you notice yourself bingeing on more carb- and fat-laden snacks when your stress triggers arise? If you're a low-hanging food grabber, have you been grabbing more "freebies" from the office cookie tray during meetings? No matter what your "type" is, be vigilant about the things that easily trip you up. Pay attention to your particular "eating type" weaknesses and monitor yourself for signs of the behaviors that have gotten you into trouble in the past.

20. Once he did, he came to a realization: He had been overweight for most of his life—and had been unhappy about it for as long as he could remember—until he found Lose It! He had worked so hard to slim down, to finally be in the best shape of his life. Was he willing to just let that go by quitting the very habit—logging his foods—that had gotten him to his goal?

"I thought to myself, 'You know what, logging my food takes only 5 minutes out of my entire day.' There's something about logging all that information that becomes a project, and you don't want all that work that you've done to be for naught."

As you might have already guessed, Brad started logging again, and pretty soon he was back on track and the 10 pounds had vanished. Now that he's in maintenance mode, he's keeping himself accountable, not to mention busy: These days, Brad's always training for a triathlon, a marathon, or another athletic challenge.

While the races he does are always changing, he says there's one thing that will always stay the same: "I'll never stop logging my calories."

FOREVER SLIM: THE TWO RULES OF MAINTENANCE MODE

After working so hard to lose the weight, you know full well how the process works. But as Brad learned, you have to remain diligent. That is why we've created the Two Rules of Maintenance Mode.

Rule # 1: Don't Stop Logging (At Least Not Right Away)

Continue logging your foods for a minimum of 3 weeks after you reach your target weight. You spent months and months adjusting to a calorie budget, and now that budget has grown. You need some time to get used to your bigger budget and to figure out what a healthy amount of "more" looks like for you. Tracking your foods for the first 3 weeks of maintenance will help you stay accountable so that you don't estimate your calorie increases or go on a Twinkie bender the moment you've been given the all-clear. And most important, you'll use those 3 weeks to gain some experience trying out your new budget, giving you the knowledge you need to develop a sense of boundaries before the training wheels come off.

During those first 3 weeks of maintenance, pay careful attention to your body's hunger and satiety signals. Ask yourself: How many calories do I feel comfortable eating? How much food can I add on a daily basis, and to which meals? How many snacks do I need? How does my increased calorie intake affect my workouts? If I decide to scale back my activity a bit, what is the impact on my weight?

During those 3 weeks, you'll have plenty of time to play around with your new budget, learning which foods and habits work for you and which ones don't. And who knows? By the end of the 3 weeks, you may just decide that the 5 minutes it takes to log your foods each day is a small price to pay for staying slim.

Rule #2: Keep Weighing Yourself

So how do you know what's working for you and what isn't?

By setting up an early warning system.

There's only one method that's been shown over and over again—by scientists and Lose It! users alike—to provide you with the best warning system. That's why Rule #2 is the ultimate red flag detector: Keep stepping on that bathroom scale.

It's best to weigh yourself regularly. This rule applies whether you're on week 3 of maintenance or year 2 of your new physique. This one small action, which takes only seconds out of your day, is hands-down one of the most crucial habits that separates people who regain weight from people who keep it off for life.

Some diets advocate avoiding the scale altogether, and some people just instinctively ignore the scale because they're worried they'll start to obsess over their weight—or they simply don't want to peer down at a number they'd rather not see.

Studies show that the more frequently you weigh yourself, the more weight you'll lose in the long run. Routinely weighing yourself allows you to monitor your weight closely, which means that if a problem arises—say you're unexpectedly taking in more calories than you thought—you'll notice immediately and make the necessary changes.

In 2009, scientists conducted a study of 3,000 members of the National Weight Control Registry, analyzing the data of people who had lost at least 30 pounds and kept it off for a minimum of 1 year. At the start of the study, nearly half of the group said they weighed themselves daily; the other half weighed themselves regularly, though not as frequently.

But not everyone kept up the habit.

At a follow-up a year later, the researchers looked at whether people had regained weight, lost it, or stayed the same, and they investigated everyone's weighing routines. Ultimately, they found that weight gain was "significantly greater" among the people who decreased the frequency with which they stepped on the scale. In other words, the people who gained the most weight were the people who paid less and less attention to the scale—regardless of whether they were initially weighing themselves

WEIGH TO GO

To make the most of your weigh-ins, you need a good scale. If you're in the market for a new one, then skip the dial types and go straight for a digital. They're more accurate, and you can find a good digital scale for as little as $35.

After their most recent tests of digital scales, *Consumer Reports* magazine ranked four at the top of its list. Rankings were based on each scale's ability to be accurate within about 1 pound of actual weight at least 97 percent of the time.

The magazine also recommended skipping the scales with body-fat indicators because most aren't very reliable and they drive up the cost of the scale.

1. **The Taylor 7506, $35.00.** This sleek, glass-and-chrome, lithium-battery-operated bathroom scale has everything you need. It scored the highest in the *Consumer Reports* test.

2. **The Tanita HS-302, $59.99.** It's double the price of the Taylor 7506, but it's also highly accurate and a favorite of the environmentally conscious because it's made from biodegradable material and has built-in solar cells.

3. **The Escali XL180, $39.95.** The Escali is accurate to within 0.2 pounds and has an extralarge display that continues showing your weight even after you've stepped off.

4. **The Tanita HD-357, $64.99.** It's not cheap, but this Tanita is light (3.5 pounds), so you can take it with you when you're traveling. It has an ultralow-profile platform (0.6 inches), making it easier to pack, and a handle, so you can carry it easily.

once every day or once every 5 days. When they started ignoring the scale, they started gaining weight.

"Consistent self-weighing," the scientists wrote, can "help individuals maintain their successful weight loss by allowing them to catch weight gains before they escalate and make behavior changes to prevent additional weight gain."

In another study published in the *American Journal of Preventive Medicine* in 2009, a team of scientists followed 100 overweight adults who enrolled in a Weigh By Day trial as part of their efforts to lose weight. After following the men and women from 2005 to 2007, the researchers found that regular self-weighing was "a significant predictor of body weight over time" and that the subjects lost about 1 extra pound for every 11 days they weighed themselves during the study period. And another study by scientists at the University of Minnesota in 2005 examined data collected from over 3,000 adults enrolled in weight-loss programs and concluded that daily weigh-ins were better than weekly weigh-ins for maintaining success.

Many people prefer to weigh themselves daily, which is fine. If you're not one of them, that's okay, too. Just make sure you're weighing yourself a *minimum* of once every 3 or 4 days.

Remember, your weight can fluctuate by as much as 3 pounds from one day to the next. If you step on the scale on Wednesday and you're 2 pounds heavier than you were on Monday, don't panic. According to Dr. Arlene Spark, an associate professor of nutrition at Hunter College in New York City, there are any number of noncalorie-related causes for the number on your scale to increase, from water retention (see page 172) to a brief illness like a cold or flu, to an increase in exercise frequency or intensity.

BUILD LOW-CALORIE RECIPES WITH LOSE IT!

Did you know that you can create new recipes using Lose It!'s recipe-building feature? You can store your recipes, alter them when you decide to change a thing or two, and even share them with your friends. Here's how.

To Create a Recipe

1. From the "My Day" screen, select the "More" tab on the bottom right.

2. Select "Edit Foods and Exercises," then click on "Recipes." The recipes screen shows you a list of your current recipes and allows you to create a new recipe.

3. Tap the icon with the plus sign to start making the recipe. Give your name a recipe and press "Save."

4. Now select the serving size. If the stir-fry you made feeds four people, then select four and press "Save." When you go to log this dish later, you can select how many servings you ate and you'll automatically get the correct nutritional information for that portion.

5. Now that you have this basic information, you can start adding ingredients to your recipe by tapping "Add Food." This brings you to the food search you're already familiar with. When you find your ingredient, select the portion and click "Add." That'll bring you back to the recipe page. Keep adding your foods until your recipe is complete.

If you see your weight increase a small amount from one day to the next, it may be nothing, says Dr. Spark. But once you get to 4 or 5 pounds of weight gain, then consider that a red flag (see page 181). It could mean you're doing something wrong. Look over your log from the previous days. Were you eating something new? Have you been going overbudget? Maybe you underestimated the calorie count of some new meals or entered some wrong serving sizes.

If you've stopped logging altogether, then now is the time to start up again and figure out where you've been spending your calories. When you see the numbers, make small changes; in a few weeks you'll be back on track.

By now you know what to look for. You know how to correct anything that's leading you astray. Visiting the scale every few days and tracking your calories as diligently as you did when you were losing all of the weight will help you keep the weight off for life. Just ask Dean and Carol Reed.

LOSING IT FOR LIFE: TWO CAN DO IT BETTER

Dean, 63, and his wife, Carol, 65, were not exactly the picture of excess, but food was a constant source of struggle in their lives.

"We always ate well, but we just ate too much and we didn't exercise enough," Carol said.

Then, in July of 2008, Carol broke her kneecap. As she dealt with a difficult and painful recovery that limited her mobility, keeping her weight under control became even more of a struggle. Carol was worried about her health; her cholesterol level had soared to an unhealthy high of 250 points. Her doctor suggested that she would soon need medication.

At 5 foot 5 and 165 pounds, Carol's body mass index fell in the overweight zone. Her husband, Dean, weighed in at nearly 220 pounds. They tried dieting together and did manage to lose a few pounds. But it wasn't until they discovered Lose It! that things really started to change.

"Our son came to visit over Christmas and he told us about a free program that helps you manage your diet and exercise," said Carol. "We have iPhones and we love them, so we downloaded Lose It! We just looked at each other and decided, we're going to do this!"

Dean said, "I had always been resistant to diets in general and kept insisting that it was all about exercise—mainly because I just didn't want to give up eating the things I like. But the breakthrough with Lose It! was that it was so easy to count calories; we just had to keep track of the foods we ate, not points or any other complicated system."

But what really made the difference for this couple was being able to clearly understand the link between calories consumed and calories burned.

"It allowed us to factor in exercise and give ourselves credit for exercise, and that allowed us to make the connection conceptually between intake and burning calories. That motivated us to exercise more, because we could see that it would offset the calories we ate," said Dean.

Dean and Carol were hugely motivated by being able to glance at their iPhones to see their daily budgets and watch in real time how their food and exercise choices were having an impact on their progress. They decided to make exercise an integral part of their lives again, as much of a routine as brushing their teeth. But they didn't overdo it. They both enjoy walking and swimming. Carol is retired, so she regularly walks 5 miles a day and mixes in swimming. Dean works full time, so he joins her for either a walk or a swim each day.

"Every night the two of us would get together after we had dinner and had exercised," says Carol. "We would enter our foods for the day and we would build new recipes (see page 187). We have a lot of custom foods and we have a lot of recipes," says Dean.

In addition to exercising regularly, Dean and Carol made some crucial changes at the dinner table. Like anyone, they both love bread and wine and cheese, but they decided to cut back a little and enjoy these foods in moderation. They still have wine every night, for example, but they limit themselves to 4 ounces most nights—going up to 8 ounces a couple of nights a week—instead of letting themselves have unlimited pours. They also go easy on the bread now, says Carol.

"If I go out to dinner and there's bread on the table, I'll eat one piece and that's it. We can have bread with dinner, but we do it in moderation."

As time went by, the weight came off. They could feel themselves getting fitter and healthier. But Dean and Carol took a conservative approach. They wanted a plan that would work for life, so they chose to lose about 0.5 to 1 pound a week over the course of a year.

"Losing the weight over a year was our choice," said Dean. "We could've lost it more quickly if we had wanted to, but we thought that it made more sense for us to do it very gradually and allow our bodies to adjust along the way. That was our strategy."

It was a strategy that worked beautifully. After using Lose It! for a year, Carol and Dean each lost 40 pounds and reached their goal weights. They've kept the weight off for a year so far, and they can see that they're not just healthier on the outside, they're healthier inside, as well. Carol, for example, has seen her cholesterol levels plummet, going from 250 all the way down to 171.

Carol's Heart-Healthy Makeover

	Before Lose It!	After Lose It!	Notes
Total Cholesterol	250	171	In general, total cholesterol should be no higher than 200.
HDL ("good") Cholesterol	46	46	HDL should be above 40.
LDL ("bad") Cholesterol	157	106	An optimal LDL level is around 100; 160 is considered high.
Ratio	5.4	3.72	An optimal ratio is between 3.5 and 5.

Dean and Carol are optimistic about the future. "We know that we have to watch what we eat and we need to exercise," said Dean, "but we're confident that we can keep the weight off."

By taking control of their food choices and their health, Dean and Carol took control of their lives. And they're not alone.

GETTING BACK ON TRACK

At 36 years old, Lose It! user Kent Metschan of Texas had a great career and a zeal for living an active life. When he wasn't working or traveling, he was always running or playing sports, even doing a triathlon. And yet, at 5 foot 7, he weighed in at an unhealthy 224 pounds.

"I wasn't superfat, but I knew my weight was affecting my health. My cholesterol was high. I have two daughters, and I thought, this is terrible. I've got to do something. My doctor told me I needed to lose 30 or 40 pounds."

Kent's issue wasn't a lack of physical activity. The problem was food:

ample portions of pizza, pasta, fast food, and desserts. Like so many Americans, Kent tried time and again to slim down on all of the popular diets, but nothing worked. Kent says he couldn't live according to someone else's meal plan.

"When you try a diet that's a complete lifestyle change, it can only last for so long," he said.

When Kent discovered Lose It!, he said, everything just clicked. He'd learned from his history of failed diet attempts not to make too many drastic changes too fast. When he began logging his foods and reviewed his log, he realized that he'd been taking in too many calories. "I thought that if I cut back my calories by 15 or 20 percent, I could weigh 15 or 20 percent less, too," he said.

At the same time, Kent took a closer look at his environment and the people around him. He thought about their eating patterns and how those patterns affected their weight.

"I have a lot of friends who aren't afraid to get a soda or eat a cheeseburger because they don't finish everything on their plate," he said. "Thinking about all that made me realize that I needed to reduce my portions."

The first thing Kent did was clean out his cupboards and get rid of the large dinner plates. "I moved to smaller plates—I ate all of my meals off of salad plates."

Then he set some self-imposed speed limits—no more rushing through his meals. He began pacing himself, allowing at least 15 minutes for his food to digest before reaching for seconds. "My whole life, I'd always be completely full after a meal, and half an hour later I'd feel miserable. I had been overeating, but I've learned to eat just until I am full."

To keep himself fuller on fewer calories, Kent also added more protein and fiber to his diet. The fixes were small, but the results were enormous: By 2010, Kent had lost more than 40 pounds.

"I weigh now what I did in high school. I spent the last 18 years in a state that was just miserable," he said. "I was almost angry when I reached my goal weight because I was like, 'I just wasted half my life, and this was so easy.'"

Kent has been in maintenance mode ever since. To maintain his new weight, he uses the same principles that helped him lose the weight in the first place. He doesn't skip meals, and he doesn't deprive himself. When he wants pizza, he eats it, but just a slice or two. And when he wants dessert, he has a modest portion.

"I know that if I don't enjoy what I'm eating, I'm not going to be able to stick to my plan and lose weight," he said.

Kent stopped logging when he went into maintenance mode, but he still weighed himself regularly. At one point he was shocked to see that some of the weight was starting to creep back on. He began diligently logging his food and exercise again, and he discovered two problems: His physical activity levels had dipped, and some of his new food choices weren't as low in calories as he'd assumed.

"One sandwich shop I go to has a California club with alfalfa sprouts, avocado, and turkey. I figured it was healthy, but after looking up the ingredients with Lose It!, I realized that it contained about 700 calories, and that's before adding in a drink. I go to that place every day—that's over 1,000 calories a day just for lunch."

After making changes to his diet and exercise program, Kent lost the weight he'd regained and is now confident that he has the tools to maintain his healthy lifestyle for years to come.

"Lose It! is the only program that's a long-term solution," he said. "It shows you how to make healthy changes that will keep the weight off for good."

REFERENCES

Chapter 1

Berg, C., A. Rosengren, N. Aires, G. Lappas, K. Torén, D. Thelle, and L. Lissner. Trends in overweight and obesity from 1985 to 2002 in Göteborg, West Sweden. *Int J Obes (Lond)*. 2005 Aug; 29(8): 916–24.

Blümel, J. E. Changes in body mass index around menopause: a population study of Chilean woman. *Menopause* 2001 Jul–Aug; 8(4): 239–44.

Bollinger B, et al. Calorie Postings in Chain Restaurants. http://www.gsb.stanford.edu/news/ StarbucksCaloriePostingStudy.pdf

Brown, W. J., L. Williams, J. H. Ford, K. Ball, and A. J. Dobson. Identifying the energy gap: magnitude and determinants of 5-year weight gain in midage women. *Obes Res*. 2005 Aug; 13(8): 1431–41.

Centers for Disease Control and Prevention (CDC). Trends in intake of energy and macronutrients—United States, 1971–2000. *MMWR Morb Mortal Wkly Rep*. 2004 Feb 6; 53(4):80–2.

Dansinger, M. L., et al. Comparison of the Atkins, Ornish, Weight Watchers, and Zone diets for weight loss and heart disease risk reduction: A randomized trial. *JAMA*. 2005 Jan 5; 293(1):43–53.

Ebrahimi-Mameghani, M., J. A. Scott, G. Der, M. E. Lean, and C. M. Burns. Changes in weight and waist circumference over 9 years in a Scottish population. *Eur J Clin Nutr*. 2008 Oct; 62(10): 1208–14.

Flegal, K. M., M. D. Carroll, C. L. Ogden, and L. R. Curtin. Prevalence and trends in obesity among US adults, 1999–2008. *JAMA*. 2010 Jan 20; 303(3):235–41.

Food Information Council Foundation, 2010 Food & Health Survey http://www.foodinsight.org/Resources/Detail.aspx?topic=2010_Food_Health_Survey_ Consumer_Attitudes_Toward_Food_Safety_Nutrition_Health

Hill, J. O. Can a small-changes approach help address the obesity epidemic? A report of the Joint Task Force of the American Society for Nutrition, Institute of Food Technologists, and International Food Information Council. *Am J Clin Nutr.* 2009 Feb; 89 (2): 477–-84.

Sacks, F. M., et al. Comparison of weight-loss diets with different compositions of fat, protein, and carbohydrates. *N Engl J Med.* 2009 Feb 26; 360(9):859–73.

Wansink B, et al. Meal size, not body size, explains errors in estimating the calorie content of meals. *Ann Intern Med.* 2006 Sep 5; 145(5):326–32.

Chapter 2

2010 Food & Health Survey. http://www.foodinsight.org/Content/3651/2010FinalFullReport.pdf

Hollis, J. F., et al. Weight loss during the intensive intervention phase of the weight-loss maintenance trial. *Am J Prev Med.* 2008 Aug; 35(2): 118–26.

National Institutes of Health, "We Can! Portion Distortion Quiz."http://www.nhlbi.nih.gov/health/public/heart/obesity/wecan/downloads/portion-quiz.pdf

Sacks, F. M., et al. Comparison of weight-loss diets with different compositions of fat, protein, and carbohydrates. *N Engl J Med.* 2009 Feb 26; 360(9): 859–73.

Wansink, B., et al. Mindless Eating: The 200 Daily Food Decisions We Overlook. *Environment and Behavior.* 2007; 39:1, 106–123.

Wyatt, H. R., et al. Long-term weight loss and breakfast in subjects in the National Weight Control Registry. *Obes Res.* 2002 Feb; 10(2):78–82.

Chapter 3

Bahr, R., and O. M. Sejersted. Effect of intensity of exercise on excess post-exercise oxygen consumption. *Metabolism.* 1991. 40(8), 836–841.

Bea, J. W., et al. Resistance training predicts 6-yr body composition change in postmenopausal women. *Med Sci Sports Exerc.* 2010 Jul; 42(7):1286–95.

Borsheim, E., and R. Bahr. Effect of exercise intensity, duration, and mode on post-exercise oxygen consumption. *Sports Medicine.* 2003. 33(14) 1037–1060.

Chad, K. E., et al. The effect of exercise duration on the exercise and post-exercise oxygen consumption. *Canadian Journal of Sport Science.* 1988. 13(4), 204–207.

Conzett-Baumann, K, et al. The daily walking distance of young doctors and their body mass index. *Eur J Intern Med.* 2009 Oct; 20(6):622–4.

Curioni, C. C., and P.M. Lourenço. Long-term weight loss after diet and exercise: a systematic review. *Int J Obes* (Lond). 2005 Oct; 29(10):1168–74.

Gibala, M. J. High-intensity interval training: a time-efficient strategy for health promotion? *Curr Sports Med Rep.* 2007 Jul; 6(4):211–3.

Healy, G. N., et al. Breaks in sedentary time: beneficial associations with metabolic risk. *Diabetes Care.* 2008 Apr; 31(4):661–6.

Jonathan, P. L., et al. A practical model of low-volume high-intensity interval training induces mitochondrial biogenesis in human skeletal muscle: potential mechanisms. *The Journal of Physiology,* 2010; DOI: 10.1113/jphysiol.2009.181743

Levine, J. A. Nonexercise activity thermogenesis—liberating the life-force. *J Intern Med.* 2007 Sep; 262(3):273–87.

Levine, J. A, et al. Non-exercise activity thermogenesis: the crouching tiger hidden dragon of societal weight gain. *Arterioscler Thromb Vasc Biol.* 2006 Apr; 26(4):729–36.

Olsen, R. H., et al. Metabolic responses to reduced daily steps in healthy nonexercising men. *JAMA.* 2008 Mar 19; 299(11):1261–3.

Perceived Exertion Scale courtesy of the CDC. www.cdc.gov/physicalactivity/everyone/measuring/index.html

Robertson, R. J., et al. Perception of physical exertion during dynamic exercise: a tribute to Professor Gunnar A. V. Borg. *Percept Mot Skills.* 1998 Feb; 86(1):183–91.

Schmitz, K. H, et al. Strength training and adiposity in premenopausal women: strong, healthy, and empowered study. *Am J Clin Nutr.* 2007 Sep; 86(3):566–72.

Talanian, J. "Interval Training Burns More Fat, Increases Fitness, Study Finds." University of Guelph (2007, June 29). *ScienceDaily.* Retrieved September 3, 2010, from http://www.sciencedaily.com /releases/2007/06/070627140103.htm

Thornton M. K., and J. A. Potteiger. Effects of resistance exercise bouts of different intensities but equal work on EPOC. *Med Sci Sports Exerc.* 2002 Apr; 34(4):715–22.

Wu, T., X. Gao, M. Chen, and R. M. van Dam. Long-term effectiveness of diet-plus-exercise interventions vs. diet-only interventions for weight loss: a meta-analysis. *Obes Rev.* 2009 May; 10(3):313–23. Epub 2009 Jan 19.

Chapter 4

Christakis, N. A., and J. H. Fowler. The spread of obesity in a large social network over 32 years. *N Engl J Med.* 2007 Jul 26; 357(4):370–9.

Gerber, B. S., et al. Mobile phone text messaging to promote healthy behaviors and weight loss maintenance: a feasibility study. *Health Informatics J.* 2009 Mar; 15(1):17–25.

Kumanyika, S. K. Trial of family and friend support for weight loss in African American adults. *Arch Intern Med.* 2009 Oct 26; 169(19):1795–804.

Patrick, K. A text message-based intervention for weight loss: randomized controlled trial. *J Med Internet Res.* 2009 Jan 13; 11(1):e1.

Perez-Pastor, E. M., et al. Assortative weight gain in mother-daughter and father-son pairs: an emerging source of childhood obesity. Longitudinal study of trios (EarlyBird 43). *Int J Obes* (Lond). 2009 Jul; 33(7):727–35.

Wadden, T. A., et al. One-year weight losses in the Look AHEAD study: factors associated with success. *Obesity* (Silver Spring). 2009 Apr; 17(4):713–22.

Chapter 5

Akbaraly, T. N., et al. Dietary pattern and depressive symptoms in middle age. *Br J Psychiatry.* 2009 Nov; 195(5):408–13.

California Center for Public Health Advocacy. Sugar-Sweetened Beverages: Extra Sugar, Extra Calories, and Extra Weight. 11 / 2009, www.publichealthadvocacy.org/PDFs/Soda_Fact_Sheet.pdf

Epel, E., R. Lapidus, et al. Stress may add bite to appetite in women: a laboratory study of stress-induced cortisol and eating behavior. *Psychoneuroendocrinology.* 2001 Jan; 26(1):37–49.

Puterman, E., et al. The power of exercise: buffering the effect of chronic stress on telomere length. *PLoS One.* 2010 May 26; 5(5):e10837.

Taylor, A. H., and A. J. Oliver. Acute effects of brisk walking on urges to eat chocolate, affect, and responses to a stressor and chocolate cue. An experimental study. *Appetite.* 2009 Feb; 52(1):155–60.

Zellner, D. A., et al. Food selection changes under stress. *Physiol Behav.* 2006 Apr 15; 87(4):789–93.

Chapter 6

Brondel, L., et al. Acute partial sleep deprivation increases food intake in healthy men. *Am J Clin Nutr*. 2010 Jun; 91(6):1550–9.

Glaros, N. M, and C. M. Janelle. Varying the mode of cardiovascular exercise to increase adherence. *Journal of Sport Behavior*. 2001; 24 (1): 42–62

Grandjean, A. C., et al. The effect of caffeinated, non-caffeinated, caloric and non-caloric beverages on hydration. *J Am Coll Nutr*. 2000 Oct; 19(5):591–600.

Harvey, A. G., and S. Payne. The management of unwanted pre-sleep thoughts in insomnia: distraction with imagery versus general distraction. *Behav Res Ther*. 2002 Mar; 40(3):267–77.

Mekary, R. A., D. Feskanich, S. Malspeis, F. B. Hu, W. C. Willett, and A. E. Field. Physical activity patterns and prevention of weight gain in premenopausal women. *Int J Obes (Lond)*. 2009 Sep; 33(9):1039–47.

Nedeltcheva, A. V., et al. Sleep curtailment is accompanied by increased intake of calories from snacks. *Am J Clin Nutr*. 2009 Jan; 89(1):126–33.

Onen, S. H., et al. Prevention and treatment of sleep disorders through regulation of sleeping habits. *Presse Med*. 1994 Mar 12; 23(10):485–9.

Romero-Corral, A., F. Lopez-Jimenez, J. Sierra-Johnson, and V. K. Somers. Differentiating between body fat and lean mass-how should we measure obesity? *Nat Clin Pract Endocrinol Metab*. 2008 Jun; 4(6):322–3.

Urban, L. E., et al. The accuracy of stated energy contents of reduced-energy, commercially prepared foods. *J Am Diet Assoc*. 2010 Jan; 110(1):116–23.

Wansink, B., K. van Ittersum, and J. E. Painter. Ice cream illusions bowls, spoons, and self-served portion sizes. *Am J Prev Med*. 2006 Sep; 31(3):240–3.

Chapter 7

Butryn, M. L., S. Phelan, J. O. Hill, and R. R. Wing. Consistent self-monitoring of weight: a key component of successful weight loss maintenance. *Obesity* (Silver Spring). 2007 Dec; 15(12):3091–6.

Linde, J. A, R. W. Jeffery, S. A. French, N. P. Pronk, and R. G. Boyle. Self-weighing in weight gain prevention and weight loss trials. *Ann Behav Med*. 2005 Dec; 30(3):210–6.

VanWormer, J. J., et al. Self-weighing promotes weight loss for obese adults. *Am J Prev Med.* 2009 Jan; 36(1):70–3.

Weiss, E. C., et al. Weight regain in US adults who experienced substantial weight loss, 1999-2002. *Am J Prev Med.* 2007 Jul; 33(1): 34–40.

ACKNOWLEDGMENTS

CHARLES

I would first like to say thank you to Brandon, Whitney, Anand, Paul, JJ, and the rest of the team at Lose It!—you help make the Lose It! vision a reality every day. I would like to thank Rebecca Gradinger and Melissa Chinchillo who got everything going and kept it going. To my wife, Megan, and our two wonderful kids, I am grateful for your support and understanding during the last year.

This book wouldn't have happened without the efforts of Julie Will and the rest of the team at Rodale, including Nancy N. Bailey, Christina Gaugler, and Aly Mostel. Thank you!

Finally, I want to thank my coauthor, Anahad, whose professionalism, intelligence, and hard work were the engine that made this book possible.

ANAHAD

First and foremost, I must thank the numerous Lose It! users who agreed to be featured in this book and generously shared their inspiring stories of weight loss—both the successes and the struggles. Without their time, their patience, and their willingness to answer my countless probing questions, this book would not have been possible. As diverse and disparate as this large group of Lose It! users may be, they all agreed to take part for the same noble reason: the hope that their experiences might inspire others to regain control of their health and find happiness in their bodies.

I would also like to thank my agent, Christy Fletcher, and everyone at Fletcher and Co. for guiding this book from its inception, especially Melissa Chinchillo and Rebecca Gradinger, whose early edits and insight were invaluable. Rebecca's fun suggestions and devotion to making this book as strong as possible were invaluable.

Thank you to Charles Teague and Whitney Klinkner for helping me pull together data and conduct interviews as the project moved forward. Charles, you could not have made my job as the writer on this project any easier. And thanks, last but not least, to Julie Will for her wonderful and lightning-quick editing, which made the book so much better. I am indebted to Julie and her team of editors and designers at Rodale for their brilliant work, which was all the more impressive because they did it in record time.

INDEX

Boldface page numbers indicate photographs. <u>Underscored</u> pages indicate boxed text.